Water for Life
Community water security

by Jeff Conant and Pam Fadem

This book is part of a larger volume, *A Community Guide to Environmental Health.*

Copyright © 2008, 2015 by Hesperian Health Guides

Hesperian encourages you to copy, reproduce, or adapt all or part of this book for non-commerical purposes, see http://hesperian.org/about/open-copyright/ for Hesperian's Open Copyright License. Contact permissions@hesperian.org to use any part of this book for commercial purposes.

Water for Life   ISBN 978-0-942364-58-3

A Community Guide to Environmental Health   ISBN 978-0-942364-56-9

Contact us at:

Hesperian Health Guides
2860 Telegraph Avenue
Oakland, California, 94609USA
tel: (1-510) 845-4507
email: *bookorders@hesperian.org*
website: *www.hesperian.org*

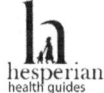
hesperian
health guides

Water for Life

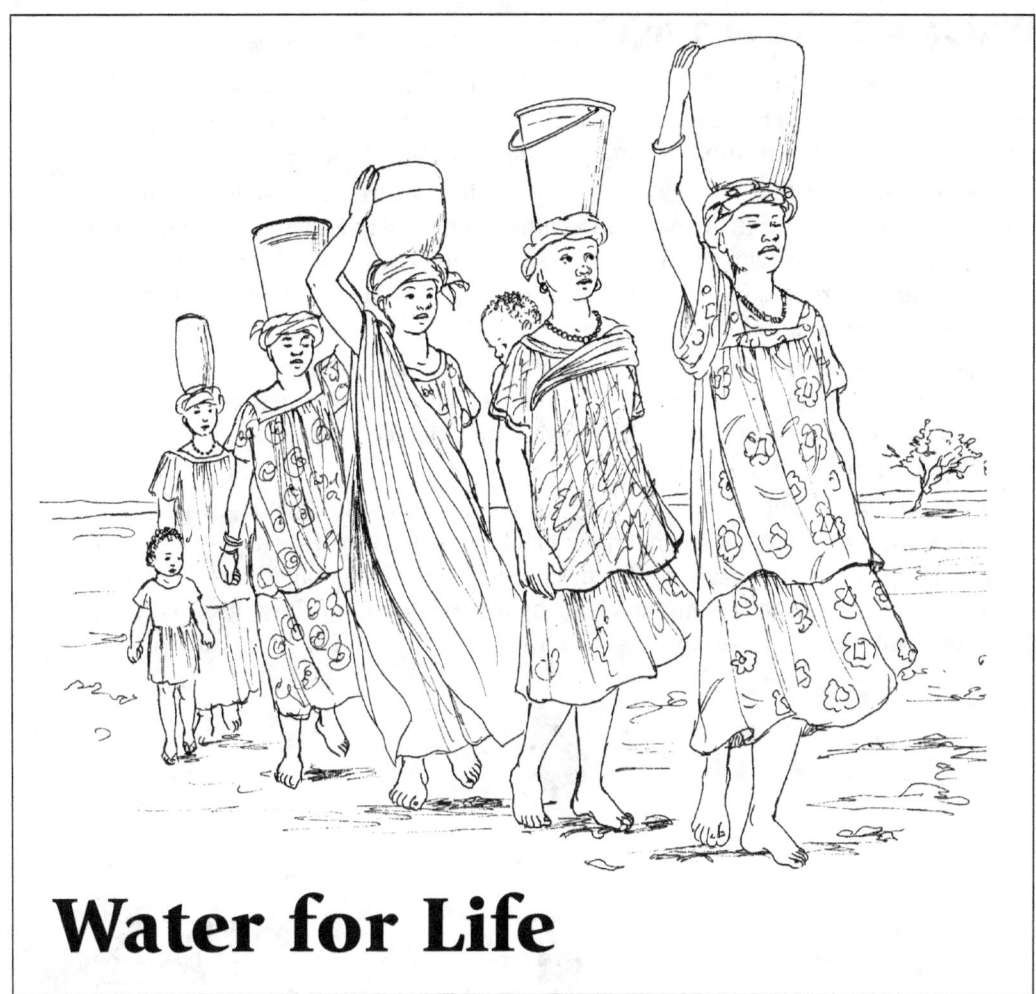

Water for Life

Water is essential for life. People, animals, and plants all need water to live and to grow. But in many parts of the world people lack enough water to stay healthy. Many people have to travel long distances to collect water. And often, the water that is available is not safe to drink.

If people do not have enough water for their daily needs, they face hardship and serious illnesses. And if the available water is not *safe* — because it is contaminated with germs, worms, or toxic chemicals — this can also lead to many illnesses.

When a community has a water supply that is *accessible* (easy to get to) and safe, everyone's health is improved. If women are freed from the daily labor of carrying and treating water, the well-being of the whole family improves. Children grow healthier and have less of the diarrhea disease that comes from contaminated water. And women and girls have more time to be part of community life and to go to school.

This booklet describes ways to collect, store, and *conserve* (save) water, and to protect and treat water so it is safe to drink. This booklet also helps to ensure *water security* (regular access to enough safe water) by raising community awareness about water problems, and by showing ways to organize for change.

The solutions offered here can be applied to small water systems anywhere. As long as all people have a say in how water is collected, conserved, and used, solutions can be found for even the most difficult problems.

Water security is a right

Because water is a basic need for all life and good health, access to enough safe water, or water security, is defined as a human right by international law. (See page 45 for more information about international laws and the right to water.)

Water is nature's gift, but there is a limit to what nature can provide. In many places the amount of water for drinking is becoming dangerously low. Where land has been paved and trees cut down, rain that once soaked into the ground and was stored as *groundwater* now runs off into the ocean and becomes salt water. Much of the water that is left is too polluted for human use.

The best way to protect our human right to water is to understand how water becomes scarce and how it is contaminated. People working together to conserve scarce water resources and share in decision making about how water is used, will ensure community water security.

Most people are willing to pay a reasonable price for safe drinking water. But in many places, water that people need for drinking is used by industry and agriculture or sold at a price people cannot afford. Whether water is managed by the community, by government, by private companies, or by a partnership of these groups, the people who need water most must have a say in how it is priced, distributed, and used.

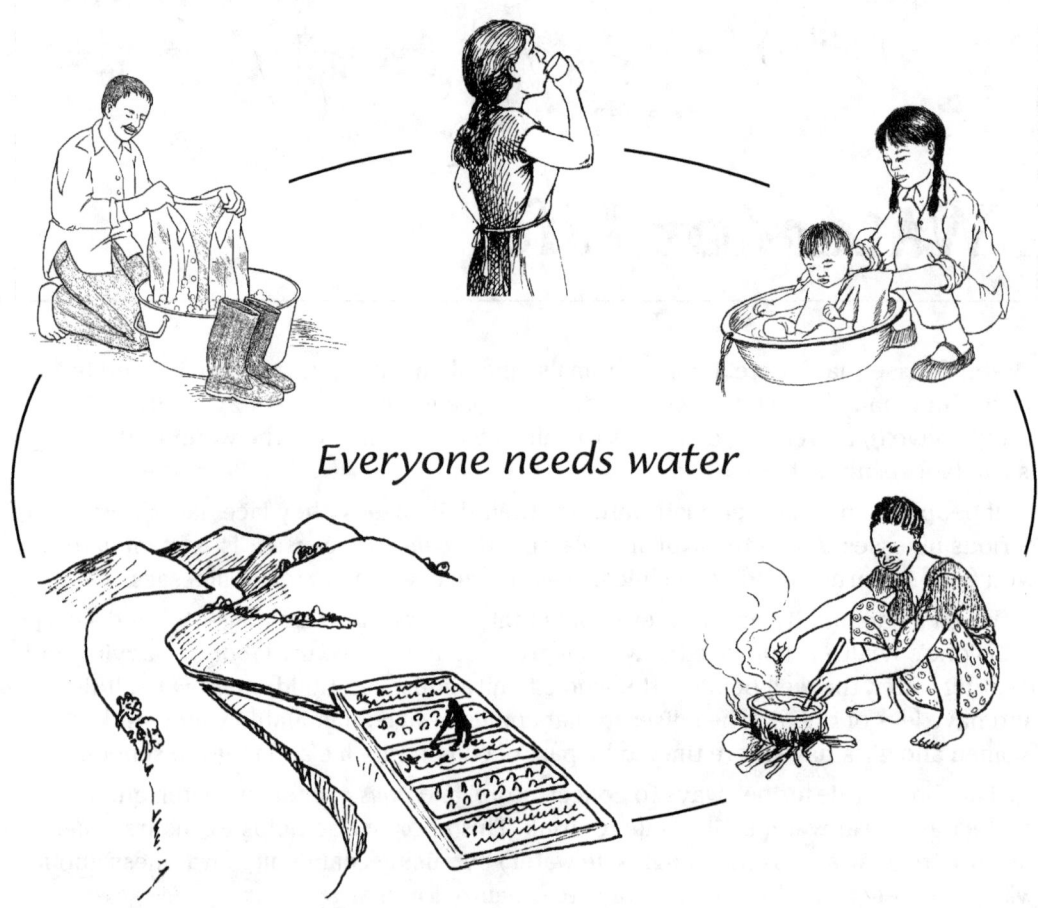

Everyone needs water

Water security improves community health

To ensure access to enough, safe water it is important to understand how to conserve, protect, store, and treat water. But understanding is not enough. The community must be motivated to change what does not work and to make these changes sustainable through community organization and action.

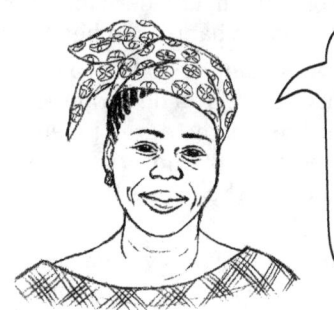

In raising community awareness, it is important to understand the root causes of problems. Many illnesses related to water security come from poverty and exploitation.

Raise community awareness of water problems

Most people already know what their problems are. A woman who carries water long distances every day does not need to be told that carrying water is hard work. But she may not feel that she has the power to make her work easier.

A community water program can create a shared understanding among a group of people. If people see water security as a community problem, they can also see that they may have the power together to make change. This is called "raising community awareness."

On the next page we share the sad story of a young boy, Timothy, who died from a lack of water security. This story is followed by the "Chain of Causes" activity. This activity may be useful to raise awareness in your community.

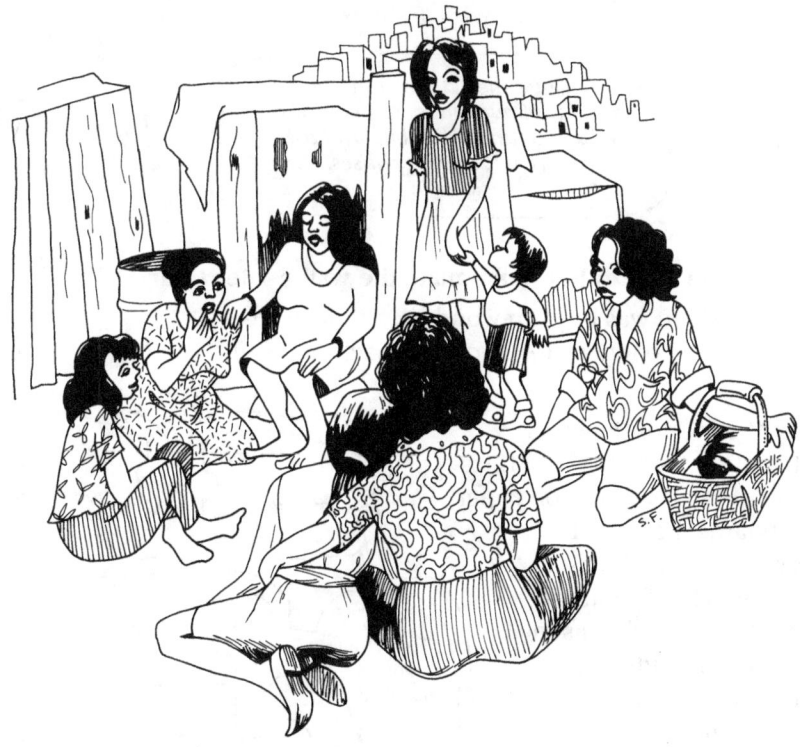

A shared understanding of a problem can help people begin to think about a shared solution.

Timothy's story

Njoki lived in the village of Luido in northern Inhambane province, Mozambique, with her young son Timothy. He was a happy and healthy child until recently.

In their village, water was pumped up from a deep tubewell. The well and pump had been built many years before by a development group. Once in a while a part of the pump would break, but 1 of the development workers always knew how to repair it or could buy a new part. But now the development workers are gone from the region. There is no one left who knows how to repair the pump, and there is no money for new parts.

When the pump broke again, Njoki's village had to rely on a water hole far from the village. The water hole, also used by many animals, was contaminated with worms, germs, and parasites. Timothy soon became very sick with severe, watery diarrhea. He became very weak and dehydrated. Njoki had no money to take her son to the health center many hours away. Within a few days, Timothy died.

But why?: Building a chain of causes

Why did Timothy die? "But why?" is a question game that helps people recognize and build a chain of causes that lead to illness and death. In this activity, ask the group for ideas about what led to Timothy's death. Each time an answer is given, ask, "But why?", helping the group to explore as many causes as possible. For example:

What caused Timothy's death? He died from diarrhea and dehydration.

But why did he have diarrhea? Because he did not have enough safe water to drink.

But why didn't Timothy's family have enough safe water?
The village pump wasn't repaired.

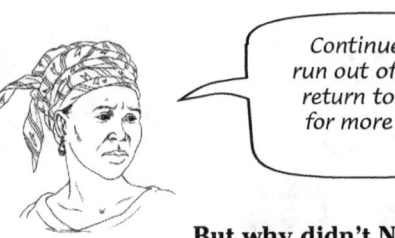

Continue the "chain" until you run out of questions. You can also return to an earlier link and ask for more underlying causes. For example:

But why didn't Njoki make the water safer to drink?
There was little firewood for boiling water and no money for *chlorine* bleach.

The "But why?" game continues as people contribute reasons for Timothy's death. A chain of causes drawn on paper or on a chalkboard, or made of cardboard or flannel, can be used to show the causes for Timothy's illness and death. For each reason given, another link is added to the chain. In this way, people can analyze the different causes of water insecurity.

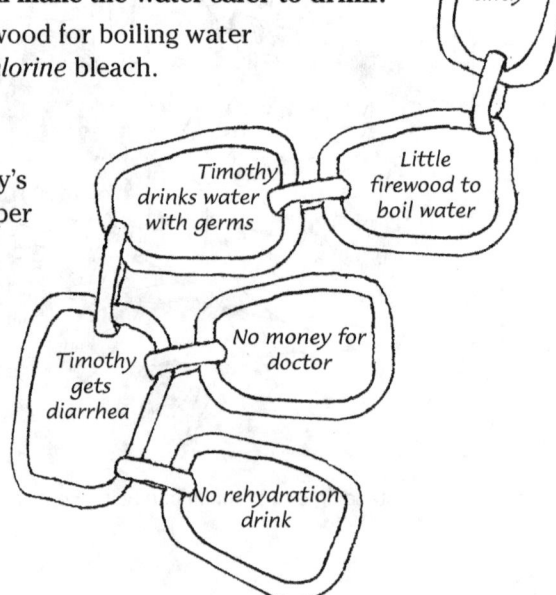

Village pump broken

Water hole far away

Little firewood to boil water

Timothy drinks water with germs

No money for doctor

Timothy gets diarrhea

No rehydration drink

Most water is used — and polluted — by industry and agriculture

Industry and farming use — and pollute — much more water than the amount used by people for their daily needs. This threatens the safety and availability of water for household use.

Because water is a human right, governments are responsible to help meet people's need for enough, safe water. It often takes people working together to make sure the government will honor and protect their rights to water security.

Industries and communities compete for water

Plachimada is a small village of rice and coconut farmers in the south of India. Farmers there have long been able to make a good living because the rainfall is plentiful and the soil is fertile. But a few years ago all of this began to change when the Coca-Cola Company built a soft drink bottling factory on the edge of the village.

The company drilled deep wells to draw up groundwater to make the cola drink. Every day the factory used 1.5 million liters of water. Villagers watched as trucks left the factory day after day, carrying away the water that once fed their crops. After the factory had been there for 2 years, villagers found that their crops were dying, their household wells had less water than before, and the water was a strange color. When they cooked rice with the water, it turned brown and tasted bad. When they drank or bathed in the water, it caused skin rashes, baldness, pain in the joints, weak bones, and nerve problems. The villagers began collecting water far from their homes to protect their health.

During a time of severe water scarcity, more than 2,000 peaceful protestors led by village women approached the Coca-Cola factory demanding that the company leave and pay the villagers for the loss of water. The company responded by sending a truckload of water to the village every day — but this was not enough to meet the villagers' needs. After 50 days of protests, police arrested 130 men and women. Many months later, 1000 people marched to the factory and again the police arrested many of them.

The struggle caused hardships for the people of Plachimada, but it also brought them together to demand their right to safe water. After several years, the local government began to support the people and ordered the company to stop using groundwater in times of drought. But the State government said the company should be allowed to continue using groundwater. The conflict went to court, where the local government supported the people of Plachimada, while the State government supported the company.

The people of Plachimada continue to suffer health problems and continue to collect water from far away. But their demand for the human right to water has received attention throughout India and the world, and their struggle has inspired many others to raise their voices. The people of Plachimada say that in a world where there is not enough safe drinking water, it makes no sense to use this precious resource to produce sweet, luxury drinks — especially if people are made sick in the process.

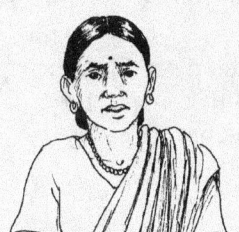

Health worker discussion questions:

• How could the company share water more fairly with the villagers?

• Does the government have a responsibility to protect people's right to water and health?

• Are there ways that your community's need for water might be better met by your local government?

Health problems from lack of water (water scarcity)

For the people who collect and carry water — usually women and children — water scarcity can mean traveling long distances in search of water. For farmers, water scarcity means hunger when drought causes crops to fail. For children, water scarcity can mean dehydration and death.

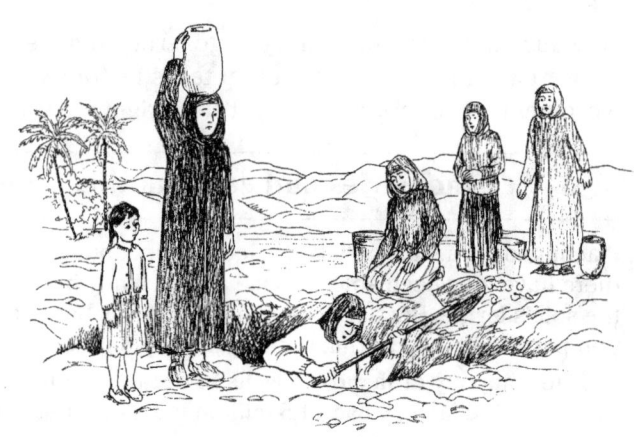

In hospitals, clinics, and other places where sick people get care, lack of water for washing can allow infection to spread from person to person. A reliable supply of safe water can mean the difference between life and death.

Collecting and carrying water over long distances causes many health problems.

Water can prevent and treat many illnesses

We need water to heal from many illnesses. Water is used to prevent and treat diarrhea. (See the book *Where There is No Doctor* and the booklet *Sanitation and Cleanliness for a Healthy Environment* for information on making a rehydration drink to treat diarrhea.) Washing hands with soap and water after using the toilet and before eating or handling food helps prevent diarrhea illnesses. If there is not enough water for washing, there is much more risk of illness and death.

How much water do we need?

People can survive much longer without food than without water. The average amount of water that 1 person needs for good health each day is:

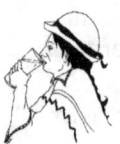

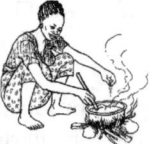

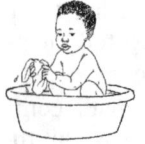

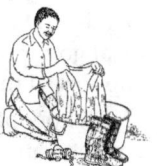

1 to 3 liters for drinking	2 to 3 liters for food preparation and cleanup	6 to 7 liters for personal cleanliness	4 to 6 liters for laundry

This totals 15 to 20 liters per person per day. But many people are forced to manage with much less. Other needs, such as sanitation, irrigation and watering livestock often require much more water than drinking, cooking and washing.

Community places such as schools and health centers may need more than the average amount of water used by one person in a household. Health centers, for example, should have at least 40 to 60 liters of water per day available for every person served.

Water and HIV/AIDS

Health problems from water scarcity or germs in water can be especially dangerous to people who are already affected by chronic or life-threatening illnesses such as HIV/AIDS. But governments and organizations in areas with high rates of HIV may be less able to meet community water and sanitation needs because they must use scarce resources to care for the HIV crisis, and because they may lose workers to the disease.

The HIV/AIDS disease is NOT passed from person to person through water. But lack of water to wash and sterilize health care instruments in hospitals and health centers can make prevention of the HIV disease more difficult.

HIV makes people more vulnerable to water-related illnesses

When people's bodily defenses are weak from HIV, diarrhea diseases are more likely to affect them and it is much harder to recover. Infants and children infected by HIV are especially vulnerable. Worms that might not be life-threatening for people who are otherwise healthy can cause pneumonia if they travel into the lungs of HIV-infected people. People taking drugs for HIV may have complications when taking other drugs to treat diarrhea and worms.

HIV compromises people's access to enough safe water

It is important for people with HIV to have access to safe drinking and washing water near the home, as well as water for gardening, raising animals, and other home-based activities. Having HIV makes access to water difficult because:

- People with HIV may be too weak to collect and carry water.
- Households headed by children or elderly people may be left out of decision making, leaving their needs for water and sanitation unmet.
- Women are the main caretakers for people with HIV as well as being heavily affected by the disease itself. When they are also responsible for collecting and treating water, the burden of work becomes too much.
- HIV leads to increased poverty because it costs money to take care of the sick and because there are fewer people working to earn money for the family. This makes it much harder to pay water fees.

Water security for people with HIV

Health workers, water and sanitation promoters, and caregivers all need training about water and sanitation-related infections and how to keep people with HIV/AIDS safe. People with HIV, their caregivers, and children, women, and elders left behind by people who have died, need to be included in planning for water projects.

When water security is respected as a human right, the most vulnerable people in the community will have their needs met and everyone will be safer and healthier.

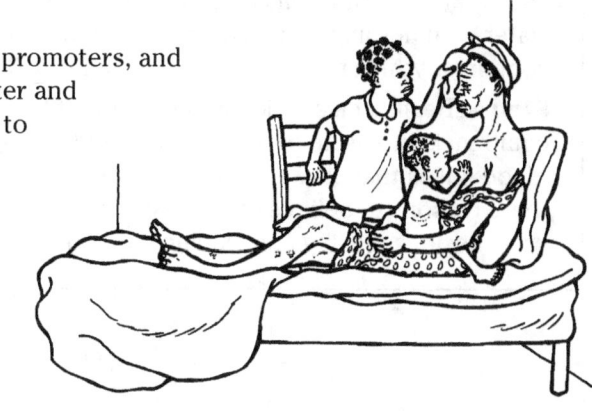

People with HIV/AIDS need safe water, good nutrition, and medicines they can afford. But most of all, they need our care and support.

Health problems from unsafe water

It can be difficult to know if water is safe or not. Some of the things that cause health problems are easily noticed by looking at, smelling, or tasting the water. Others can only be found by testing the water (see page 11). Understanding what makes water unsafe and taking steps to protect water from contamination can prevent many problems from unsafe water.

HOW DO YOU KNOW IF WATER IS SAFE?

This activity can help people understand that there may be something harmful in the water even if it cannot be seen. Because germs and toxic chemicals are often invisible, it is difficult to know what water is safe for drinking.

Time: 15 to 30 minutes

Materials: 4 clear bottles, mud, salt, sugar, treated water

Step 1: Before the activity, fill 4 clear bottles with water that has been boiled, treated with chlorine, or had some other treatment. To one bottle, add a spoonful of mud. To another, add a spoonful of sugar. To another, add a spoonful of salt. Shake the bottles well. Leave the last bottle as it is. Bring these bottles to the group.

Step 2: Ask people in the group to smell the water in all the bottles. Then invite them to drink water from any of the bottles. Most likely no one will drink the muddy water, but many will drink from the other bottles.

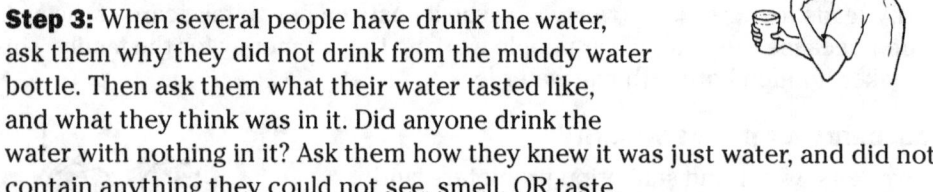

Step 3: When several people have drunk the water, ask them why they did not drink from the muddy water bottle. Then ask them what their water tasted like, and what they think was in it. Did anyone drink the water with nothing in it? Ask them how they knew it was just water, and did not contain anything they could not see, smell, OR taste.

Step 4: Begin a discussion about different things that may be in your water that could make it unsafe to drink. This could include germs that cause diarrhea, blood flukes that cause *schistosomiasis*, and pesticides or other chemicals. Are there reasons to believe that these things may be in the water? Are there other ways besides looking and smelling to know if the water is safe?

Testing for water safety

Testing water in a laboratory or with a water quality test kit can show the type and amount of contamination. Water testing may be done by professionals, who take samples of local water to a laboratory to test it. Laboratory testing is usually necessary to find chemical contamination. These tests are helpful, but can be costly.

Testing water for germs may be done locally using a test kit. One kind of test kit, called the H2S test, is widely used to test for germs in water. It is not costly (5 tests cost about 1 dollar) and it gives quick results. But this test sometimes mistakes harmless living things for germs, and it does not show if chemicals or harmful *parasite*

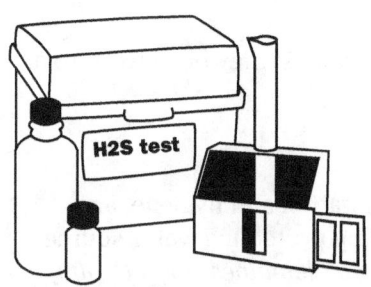

eggs are present. Another problem with this and other water quality tests is that they only show if the water is contaminated at the time and place the water sample is taken.

Water quality testing has many advantages and can be used successfully under some conditions. But it is not a replacement for a community water assessment plan, careful protection of water sources, and common sense.

Diarrhea diseases

Diarrhea, dysentery, *cholera,* and *typhoid* are caused by many kinds of germs carried by human waste, unsafe water, flies and insects, and on food. Diarrhea can be a sign of some kinds of worm and parasite infections. These illnesses may also be caused by poor sanitation and a lack of enough water for personal cleanliness.

Signs of diarrhea diseases

The most common sign of a diarrhea disease is frequent, watery stools. It may be accompanied by fever, headache, trembling, chills, weakness, and vomiting. Because there are many causes of diarrhea and dysentery, knowing what treatment to give depends on the kind of diarrhea.

These signs can help you know which diarrhea disease a person has:

- **Cholera:** diarrhea like rice water, severe intestinal pain and cramping, vomiting
- **Typhoid**: fever, severe intestinal pain and cramping, headache, constipation or diarrhea
- **Giardia:** diarrhea that appears greasy, floats and smells bad, gas and burps that smell like rotten eggs
- **Bacterial dysentery (Shigella):** bloody diarrhea, fever, severe intestinal pain and cramping
- **Amebic dysentery:** bloody diarrhea, fever, severe intestinal pain and cramping

Treatment for diarrhea diseases

Diarrhea is best treated by giving plenty of liquids and food. In most cases, no medicine is needed. These diarrhea diseases need special treatment:

- Amebic dysentery may be best treated with antibiotics. To know which antibiotics to use, see a health worker or a general health book like *Where There is No Doctor*.
- Typhoid is best treated by antibiotics because it can last for weeks and even months and lead to death.
- Cholera is best treated with rehydration drink, lots of fluids, and easy-to-digest foods to replace nutrients lost through diarrhea and vomiting. Antibiotics should only be used in the most severe cases.

If a person has bloody diarrhea, or a high fever, or is very sick, they need to go to a health center.

To prevent diarrhea and dysentery

Because most diarrhea diseases are related to poor sanitation and hygiene, and contaminated water and food, they are best prevented by protecting water sources and improving sanitation. (See the booklet *Sanitation and Cleanliness for a Healthy Environment* for information about diarrhea prevention through safe, healthy community sanitation.)

- Do not use water from unprotected sources.
- Make water safe to drink by filtering or treating it (see pages 37 to 43).
- Use toilets and wash hands after use.
- Wash hands with soap and water before handling food.
- Cook food well and protect food from germs.
- Clean baby bottles and eating utensils with boiling water to kill germs.

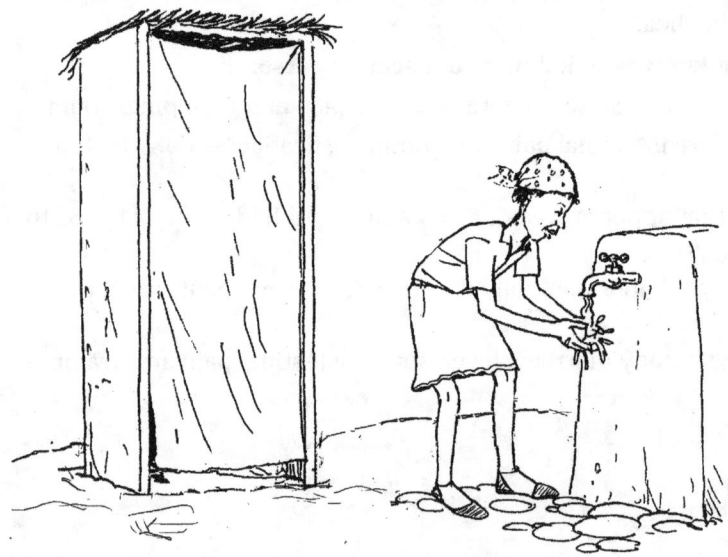

A way to wash hands close to toilets can prevent many cases of diarrhea.

Worm infections

Some worms and other *parasites* (tiny animals) that live in surface water can get into people's intestines and cause diseases. The larger ones can be seen, but most cannot. Stepping into or washing with contaminated water, drinking this water, or eating uncooked shellfish or plants can pass these worms and parasites to people.

To prevent worm infections
- Reduce contact with contaminated water.
- Keep animal waste out of water.
- Use toilets and wash hands after use.
- Cook food well and protect food from germs.
- Trim fingernails and wash hands often.
- Wear shoes to prevent worms from entering through the feet.
- Settle, filter, and disinfect drinking water.

Guinea Worm

Guinea worm is a long, thin worm that lives under the skin and makes a painful sore on the body. The worm, which looks like a white thread, can be over a meter long. Guinea worm is found in parts of Africa, India, and the Middle East.

Signs of guinea worm:
- A painful swelling develops on the ankle, leg, or elsewhere on the body.
- After a few days to a week a blister forms which soon bursts open and forms a sore. This often happens when standing in water or bathing. The end of a white thread-like guinea worm can be seen poking out of the sore. The worm works its way out of the body over the next week.
- If the sore gets dirty and infected or if the worm is broken by trying to pull it out, the pain and swelling spread and walking becomes impossible.

Guinea worm is spread from person to person like this:

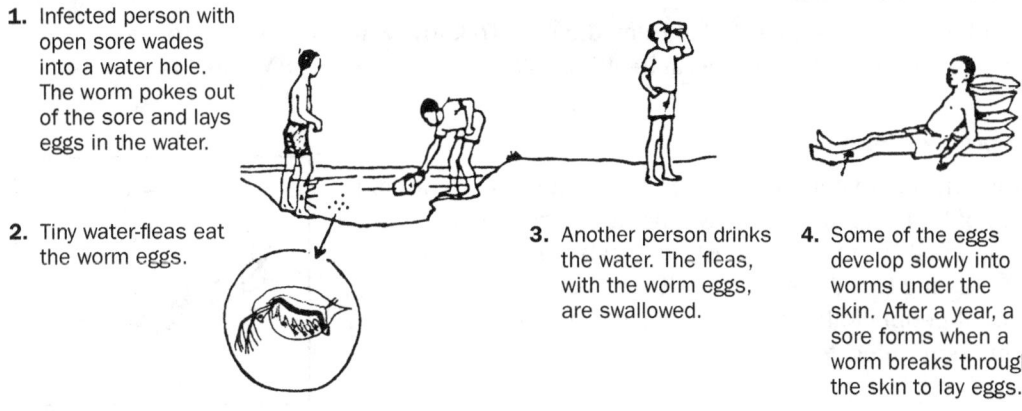

1. Infected person with open sore wades into a water hole. The worm pokes out of the sore and lays eggs in the water.

2. Tiny water-fleas eat the worm eggs.

3. Another person drinks the water. The fleas, with the worm eggs, are swallowed.

4. Some of the eggs develop slowly into worms under the skin. After a year, a sore forms when a worm breaks through the skin to lay eggs.

To treat guinea worms see a health worker or a general health book like *Where There is No Doctor*. In addition, measures should be taken to prevent new contact with worms.

To prevent guinea worms see page 23, Steps to safer water holes and page 39, Cloth filters.

Blood flukes (Schistosomiasis, bilharzia)

This infection is caused by a kind of worm that gets into the bloodstream after washing or swimming in contaminated water. The illness can cause serious damage to the liver and kidneys, and may lead to death after months or years.

Sometimes there are no early signs. A common sign in some areas is blood in the urine or bloody stools. In areas where this illness is very common, people with only mild signs or belly pain should be tested.

Blood flukes spread like this:

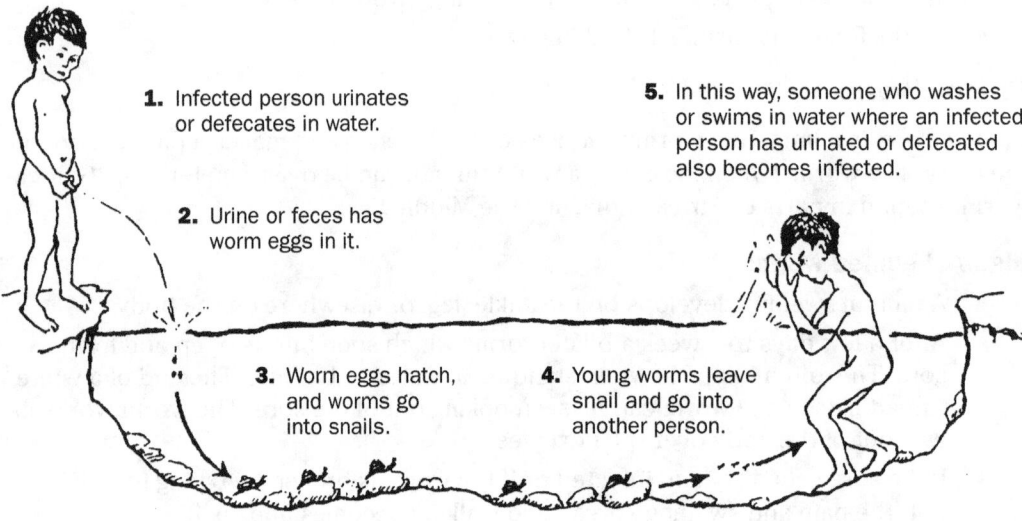

1. Infected person urinates or defecates in water.

2. Urine or feces has worm eggs in it.

3. Worm eggs hatch, and worms go into snails.

4. Young worms leave snail and go into another person.

5. In this way, someone who washes or swims in water where an infected person has urinated or defecated also becomes infected.

To treat blood flukes

Blood flukes are best treated with medicines. To know which medicines to use, see a health worker or a general health book like *Where There is No Doctor.*

To prevent blood flukes

Blood flukes do not spread directly from person to person. Part of their life they must live inside a certain kind of small water snail. To prevent schistosomiasis, programs can be established to kill these snails. These programs can only work if people follow the most basic preventive step: never urinate or defecate in or near water.

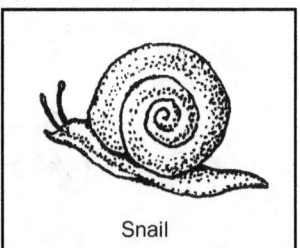

Snail

Toxic chemicals in water

Factories that produce food products, textiles, plastics, pharmaceuticals, cosmetics, and pesticides all release chemical waste into water sources. This makes the water unsafe to drink or to use for bathing or irrigation. These chemicals are usually invisible and very difficult to detect.

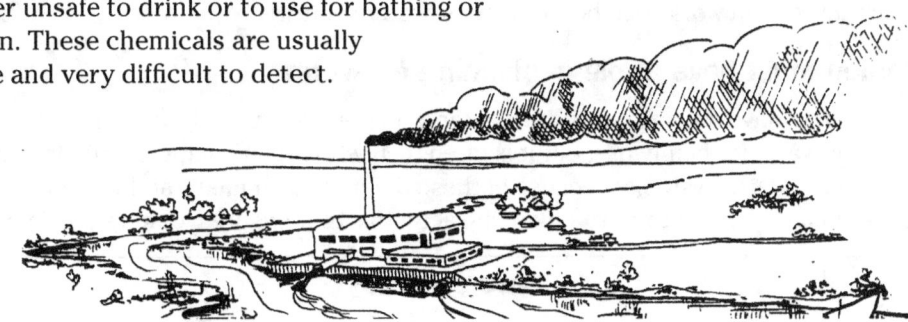

Toxic chemicals can enter the water in many ways.

The only way to know what chemicals are in the water is to test it at a laboratory. And the only way to ensure that water is free of toxic chemicals is to prevent chemical contamination at the source. To prevent contamination from toxic chemicals:

- Factories should take responsibility for treating their wastes.
- Industries like mining and oil drilling should not be done in places where water is at risk.
- Governments should set standards to prevent industrial pollution of water sources and ensure that these standards are enforced.
- Farmers who use pesticides and fertilizers should use them in limited amounts and ensure that these chemicals do not enter water sources.

Arsenic in Bangladesh

Some toxic chemicals exist naturally in the earth. When these chemicals enter our drinking water they can be deadly. This is very rare, but as water becomes scarce the risk of natural toxins grows.

The worst case of water poisoning from naturally occurring toxic chemicals was in Bangladesh in 1983. Many people started getting very ill with problems like skin lesions, cancer, nerve damage, heart disease and diabetes, and many were dying. It was one of the largest public health disasters the world had ever seen — and no one knew what was causing it.

In 1993, scientists learned that the cause of the illnesses was arsenic, a toxic chemical that was in the drinking water. Many years before, the government and international agencies had built thousands of tubewells in Bangladesh to provide safe drinking water. Before the arsenic poisoning, most people drank surface water, often contaminated with germs that led to death from diarrhea and other diseases. When the tubewells were built, nobody knew that water should be tested for arsenic.

Today there are many programs in Bangladesh to prevent poisoning by providing special water filters and new arsenic free water sources. But what could have been done to prevent the poisoning in the first place? The mystery is still not solved. Was the poisoning of so many people accidentally caused by a development project intended to save lives? The answer is not simple. The only way to prevent poisoning from toxic chemicals is to know what is in the water naturally, and to prevent any activity that may poison the water.

See page 47, Where to get more information, for a low-cost method to remove arsenic from water.

Developing a plan for community water security

When people have raised community awareness about the problems they face in meeting their water security needs (see page 5), they are ready to take the next step. Communities can work together to plan for water security.

Women must have a role in planning for water

Women may have different needs for water than men. It is usually women who collect and treat water for family use, but it is often men who are in charge of building and maintaining water systems. Because of these differences in men's and women's work and needs, it can be useful to create planning activities that ensure women's participation.

TWO CIRCLES

This activity helps women think about their water needs and the barriers they face in meeting these needs.	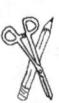	**Time:** 45 minutes to 1 hour **Materials:** Large drawing paper, drawing pens

Step 1: Divide into groups of no more than 10 people each. Give each group drawing pens and paper.

Step 2: Each group draws 2 circles on their paper, a large circle with a smaller circle inside.

Step 3: Each person draws inside the larger circle the water, sanitation, and health-related problems that affect the whole community. Inside the smaller circle they draw the problems that affect women in particular. If a person cannot draw, she can write down her thoughts.

Step 4: Now bring all the groups together into one large group and begin a discussion.

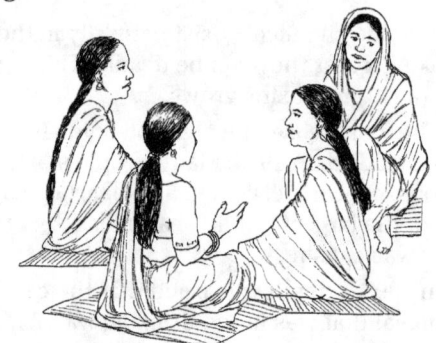

- How do the problems in the 2 circles differ?
- How are the problems similar?
- What solutions can be found for both, making sure that the women's problems receive sufficient attention?

This activity can also be done with men. Have one of the groups consist only of men, and have each group draw 2 small circles rather than only one. One of the smaller circles represents problems that affect women in particular and one represents problems that affect men.

When the groups come back together, ask the men to consider how they can help improve conditions in the community by addressing some of the issues that affect women. This may include building toilets closer to homes, carrying water, spending more time with children, and so on. It may be more comfortable to have the women discuss their issues in private before the men discuss theirs, especially in communities where men and women may have strong differences of opinion.

A Water Watch to assess community water security

A Water Watch activity can help a group choose the best sources of safe drinking water. It can also help find sources of contamination now, or possible problems in the future.

A Water Watch activity can be a long process that involves the whole community and includes many of the steps in planning a water project, or it can be a shorter process done by a small group responsible for community water safety and supply. The most important thing is to listen closely to the whole community, especially those who collect and treat water every day.

How to do a Water Watch activity

1. Talk to people who use and care for the water

Is there a person or group in the community responsible for wells, pipes, or other water supply systems? Is there a person or group responsible for sanitation? Which people or groups most often collect, carry, treat, and store the water? These people or groups should be involved in the Water Watch and in any improvements to water sources.

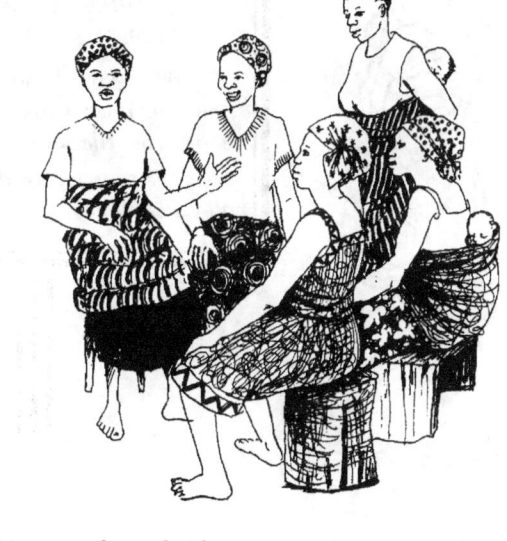

Together with the people responsible for the water, list all the water sources in the area. Note what people say about drinking water quality and quantity. Note the work it takes to collect water and ensure that it is safe, and how much time people spend doing this work.

You can ask questions like: How much water is used every day? Are different sources used for drinking, cooking, bathing, watering livestock, farming, and other needs? Is there enough water for all these needs? Is there a water source or any water storage for emergencies?

2. Make a map of local water sources and sources of contamination

A map of the community can show where the water sources are in relation to people's homes and to sources of contamination. A map should also show important landmarks such as roads, paths, houses and other buildings, farms, fields, toilets and sewer lines, and dumping sites.

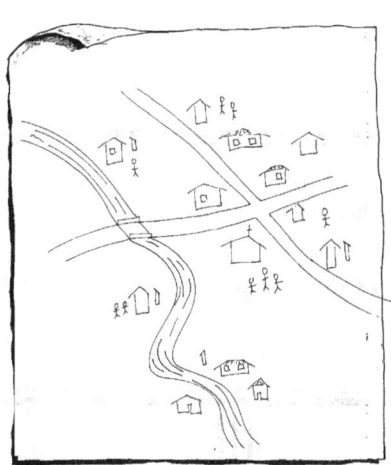

Community map

3. Visit all the places where people collect water

Different kinds of water sources can have different problems and different solutions. Visit springs, wells, *surface waters* (rivers, streams, lakes, and ponds), and rainwater catchment sites. At each water source, start a discussion about how this water is used and if anyone suspects that it is contaminated.

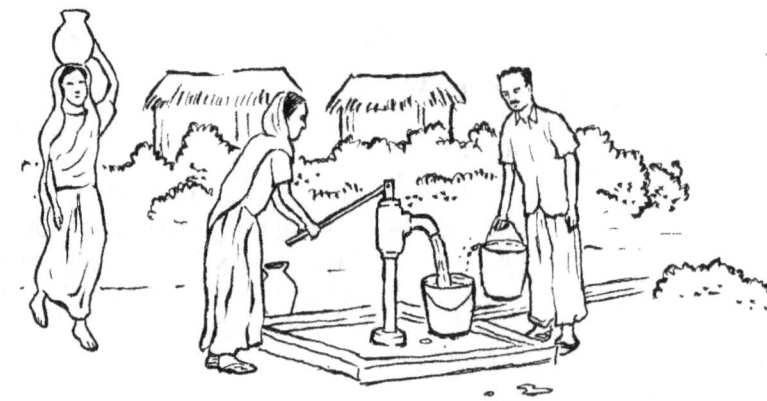

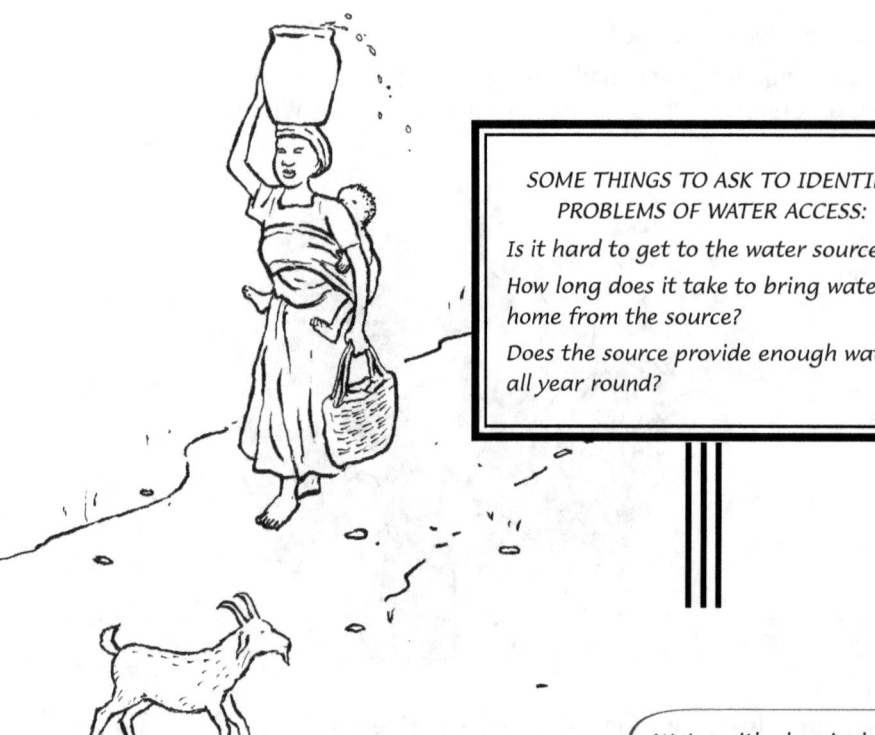

> *SOME THINGS TO ASK TO IDENTIFY PROBLEMS OF WATER ACCESS:*
>
> *Is it hard to get to the water source?*
>
> *How long does it take to bring water home from the source?*
>
> *Does the source provide enough water all year round?*

Soap does not lather well in water that contains certain minerals, making it harder to clean clothes.

Water with chemicals makes food taste bad. Rice turns brown and soft when cooked in water with high amounts of lead or other metals.

Beans do not cook well in water with a lot of minerals and salt, but the water may be safe to drink.

> *SOME THINGS TO ASK TO IDENTIFY PROBLEMS OF WATER QUALITY:*
>
> *Is the water cloudy or dirty?*
>
> *Is the water a strange color, such as red or black?*
>
> *Are there problems cooking with the water?*
>
> *Are there problems washing with the water?*

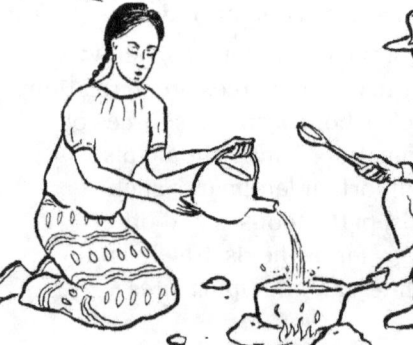

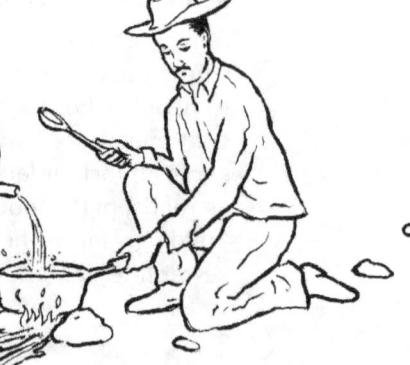

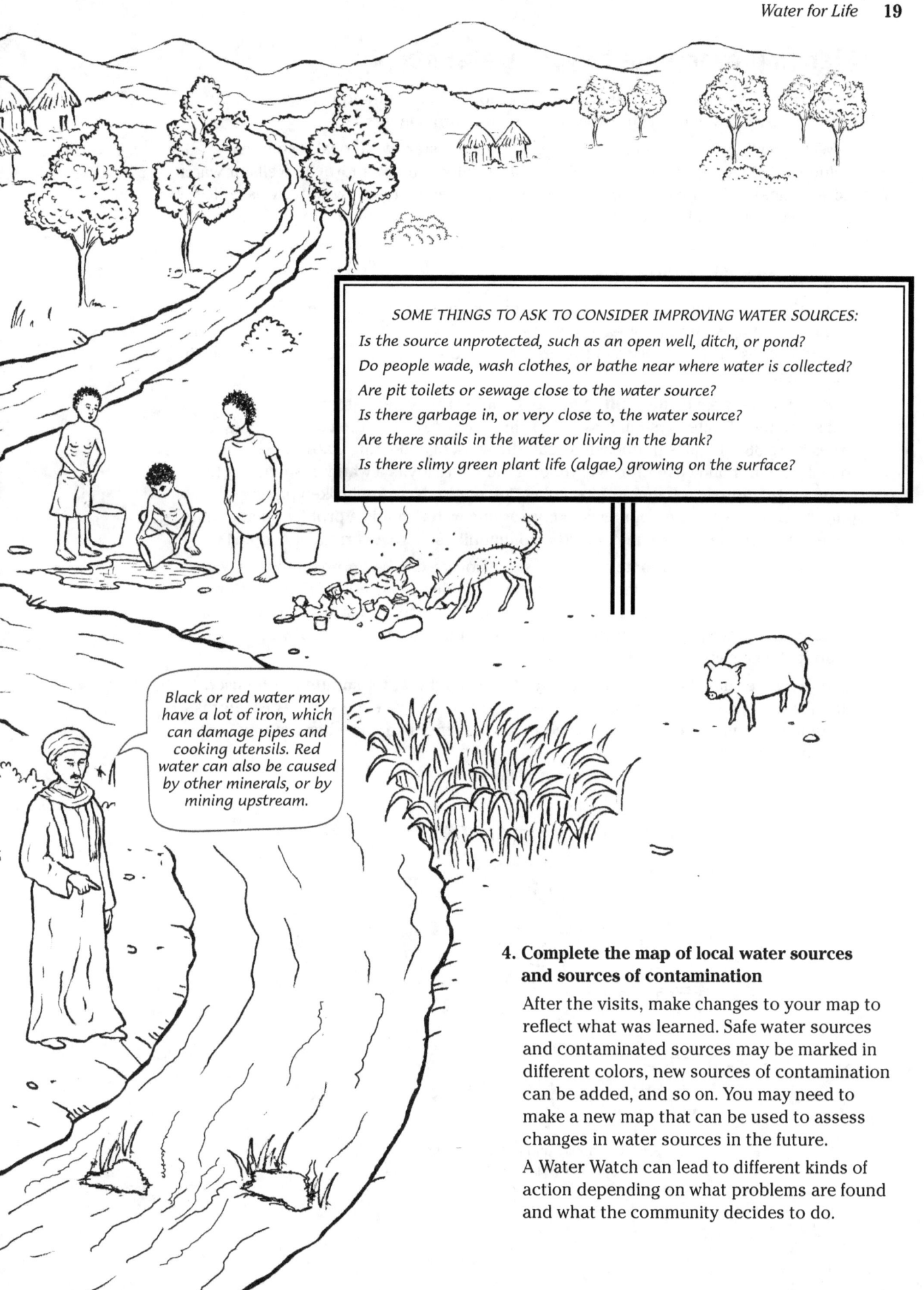

SOME THINGS TO ASK TO CONSIDER IMPROVING WATER SOURCES:

Is the source unprotected, such as an open well, ditch, or pond?

Do people wade, wash clothes, or bathe near where water is collected?

Are pit toilets or sewage close to the water source?

Is there garbage in, or very close to, the water source?

Are there snails in the water or living in the bank?

Is there slimy green plant life (algae) growing on the surface?

Black or red water may have a lot of iron, which can damage pipes and cooking utensils. Red water can also be caused by other minerals, or by mining upstream.

4. Complete the map of local water sources and sources of contamination

After the visits, make changes to your map to reflect what was learned. Safe water sources and contaminated sources may be marked in different colors, new sources of contamination can be added, and so on. You may need to make a new map that can be used to assess changes in water sources in the future.

A Water Watch can lead to different kinds of action depending on what problems are found and what the community decides to do.

Plan improvements to your water supply

After doing a Water Watch or using other methods to understand your community water security problems, you can begin to plan improvements.

When making a plan to improve the water supply, start with local resources including: local water sources, people with the skills to build improved wells or water storage tanks or install pipes, or older people who remember how water was collected many years ago. It is best to improve existing water sources before trying to develop new ones.

Identify possible solutions

The actions your community takes to improve water security depend on which problems are most urgent, or easiest to solve first. What is important is to make a plan that addresses the root causes of the problems and satisfies the needs of everyone in the community.

If water is scarce or difficult to get to, building rainwater catchment tanks, storage tanks or a piped water system may help bring water closer to the community (see pages 30 to 36). If this is not possible, can the work of collecting water be shared to make it fairer and easier for everyone? If there already is a water system, can the community improve it by improving collection methods, fixing broken pipes and pumps, protecting water sources and conserving water? If it is a problem that should be resolved by the government, can the community solicit government support?

If the water is contaminated by germs, the source can be improved or the water can be treated to make it safe. The community can discuss which of these options will be easiest, most effective, and most sustainable over time. To learn about improving water sources, see pages 22 to 29. To learn about different methods for water treatment, see pages 37 to 43.

If the water may be contaminated by chemicals the water **should not be used** until a water quality test can be done (see page 11). If a test shows that the water is contaminated, more contamination should be prevented and another water source should be developed.

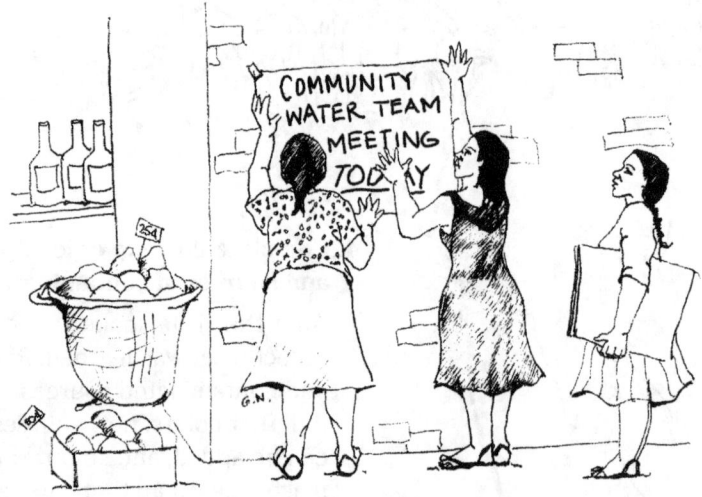

Health workers and water safety promoters can
help the community improve water security.

What are the barriers to planning a water project?

There may be many reasons why a community lacks safe water. Problems might include lack of money, lack of knowledge about building water systems, lack of support from the government, or lack of participation by people in the community. To achieve the goal of safe water, the barriers must be identified and removed one by one.

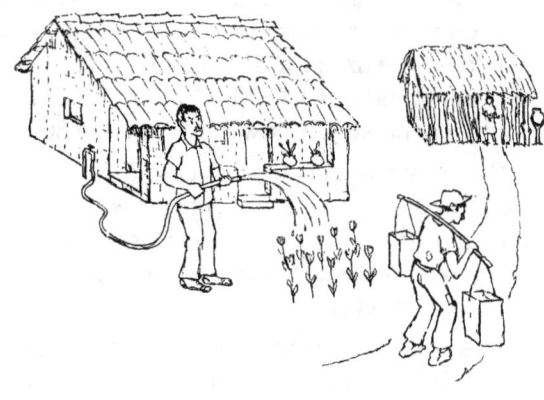

A water project should benefit everyone in the community equally.

People are more likely to improve their water source and to maintain a water system when they see:

- immediate community benefits such as more water, easier access, or less disease.
- low cost.
- only small changes in daily routine.
- positive results such as less mud, fewer mosquitoes, or more water for home gardens.

Solutions exist within the community

Throughout history, every culture has developed ways of finding and protecting water. People have used divining rods, invented devices for lifting and transporting water, planted trees to attract rain, and made laws to encourage neighboring tribes and villages to share water, prevent conflicts, and preserve this precious resource for future generations.

Villagers teach development workers

A group of development workers came to a Colombian mountain village to help the villagers fight diarrhea by protecting their water sources. When they visited the village spring, they saw that cattle and soil erosion affected the spring. The development workers suggested two simple solutions- to put up a barbed wire fence to protect the spring, or to graze their cattle elsewhere.

The villagers did not like these ideas. They predicted that the barbed wire would be stolen before long, and they did not have enough land and money to make proper cattle pastures. But seeing the problem, they came up with a solution that would work. Everyone from the village came out to plant prickly vegetation upstream from the spring. This forced the cattle to drink water at lower places along the river and solved the problem.

How to protect groundwater sources

Many people rely on water from rivers, streams, lakes, and ponds (*surface water*) as their only source of drinking water. Because surface water is often contaminated, it should not be used for drinking unless it is treated first (see pages 37 to 43 for water treatment methods.) The best alternatives to surface water are to use groundwater or to collect and store rainwater (see page 30.)

Groundwater may be collected from many kinds of wells and boreholes. Groundwater is usually free of germs because it is filtered when it seeps through sand and soil. However, groundwater can be contaminated by natural minerals such as arsenic, by leaking sewer pipes, septic tanks or latrines, by waste dumps, or by industrial chemicals.

The most serious threats to groundwater are poorly built sanitation systems, waste disposal, deforestation, overgrazing, industrial pollution, and overuse.

The best way to protect groundwater or surface water is to protect the entire area where water collects, called the *catchment area*. After a water source is developed, more people tend to gather in the area, making it harder to protect the catchment area. In places with industrial activity, water may be overused or polluted and the people who need it most may not have the power to prevent the problem. Both of these problems can only be solved through community organizing and community partnerships with government or private agencies (see pages 4 to 6 and page 44).

Different kinds of wells

There are many different kinds of wells for raising groundwater. The simplest is a hand-dug water hole, sometimes called a scoophole. The most costly kind of well, called a tubewell, is a narrow pipe going deep into the ground with a pump at the top.

The best well for any community depends on the depth of the groundwater and the resources available for digging, drilling, and building a well. But a well is only useful if people can get water out of it. For this reason, simple, shallow wells where people draw water in buckets may often be better than costly deep wells that require pumps. Before digging a well make sure that the kind of well you dig is the best for everyone's needs.

To determine if the water in any kind of well is unsafe, look for:

- pit toilets, sewer pipes, garbage dumping pits or livestock within 30 meters of the well.
- industrial activity such as mining, oil drilling, or waste dumping nearby that may affect the groundwater.
- wastewater or surface runoff getting into the well.
- Do people stand on the lip of the well or use unclean buckets when they draw water?

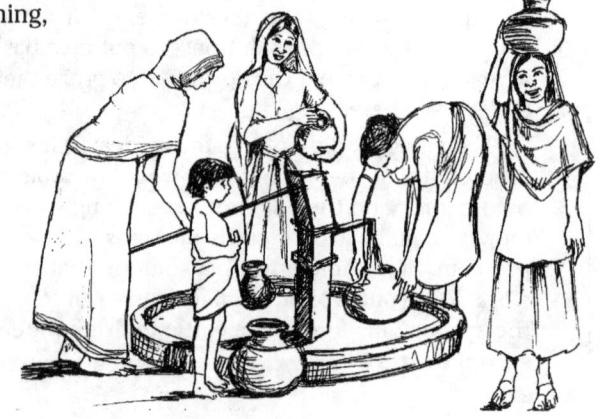

Steps to safer wells and water holes

Shallow hand-dug wells can provide good, safe water. But the water can dry up or be easily contaminated. During rainy periods, runoff water may drain into a water hole, carrying germs and other contamination. The muddy conditions around water holes make it easy for germs to collect on the feet of people or animals that use the water. Buckets and ropes around the rim of the well may also collect germs and can easily contaminate the water when they are lowered into the well.

Making simple improvements can prevent contamination. One improvement is to ensure that only clean buckets and ropes are lowered into the water. Building up earth around the hole or lining the top with bricks or concrete rings will also make the water safer. Lining the hole has the additional benefit of making it less likely to dry up or collapse.

Before drilling new wells or making costly improvements to water systems, consider making small improvements like these to make your water sources safer.

Improvements to open water holes

Build stone steps into the water hole so people can draw water from the last step without getting wet. Always use the last dry step. Never wade into the water.

Or turn the water hole into a well so people can draw water with a clean rope and bucket.

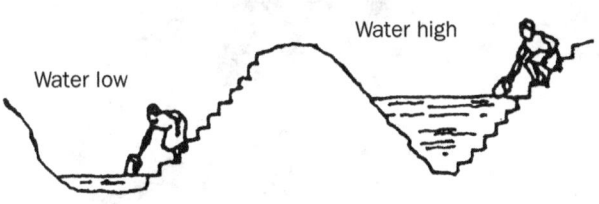

Water high

Water low

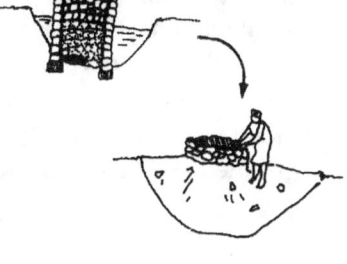

Improvements to basic wells and scoopholes

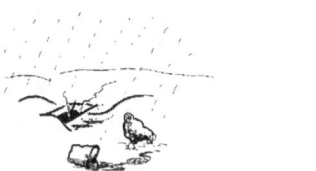

1. Unimproved scoophole

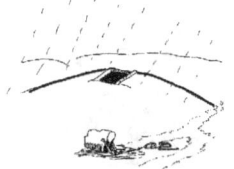

2. Mouth of hole built up to keep out runoff

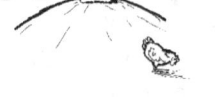

3. Mouth closed off with barrel and lid

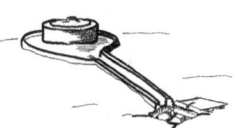

4. Top strengthened with bricks and small drainage platform

5. Protected water hole with drainage platform and runoff channel

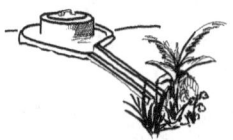

6. Protected water hole with drainage platform, runoff channel, and garden

> **IMPORTANT**   Never drink directly from a water hole. Filtering the water and letting it settle will remove some germs. Water treatment methods are described on pages 37 to 43.

The protected family well

Many communities have tubewells built for them by governments and international agencies. One reason for making these wells is to better protect the water from contamination by people and animals. But 4 to 5 years after they are drilled, many of these wells can no longer be used because the pumps break, spare parts are no longer available, or the people who can fix them are gone. This can lead to water insecurity. In some parts of Africa, tubewells are now being replaced by "protected family wells" that protect water quality and ensure water security.

Where to dig a well

The best sign that there will be water is other wells nearby. But if they are deep boreholes this may mean the groundwater is too deep to get to by hand digging. Another good sign is the year-round presence of plants that need a lot of water to survive. Low areas are more likely to have water than higher ground. But if a well is dug in a low area it will need to be protected from rainwater runoff.

To make a protected family well

A protected well has a lining, a concrete cover slab, a *windlass*, and a drainage platform. Each one of these things adds some measure of protection to the well. With all of them in place, and with careful handling of the water, a well can be considered very safe.

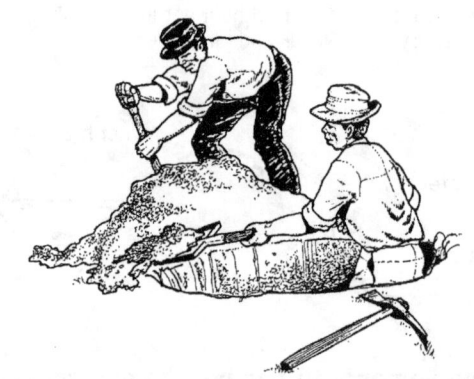

Digging a well and making a lining is difficult and dangerous. It is best done by trained and experienced well diggers.

The well lining

Traditional wells often have no lining. In very firm soils, lining the well may seem unnecessary. But it is wise to line at least the top 1½ to 2 meters below ground to prevent the side walls from collapsing. If the entire well is lined, it will make the water source more dependable, but it will be more difficult to dig the well deeper at a later time. A well can be lined with stones or rocks, with fired bricks, or with concrete.

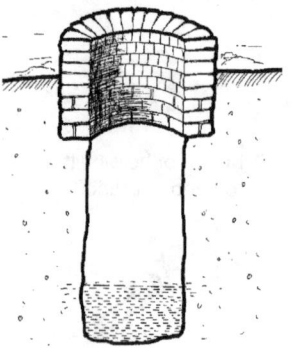

Top 1 ½ to 2 meters lined

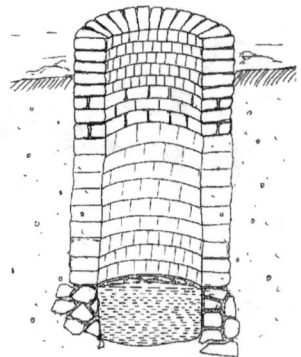

Fully lined well

HOW TO MAKE A COVER SLAB

Once a well has been lined, the next stage of protection is fitting a concrete cover slab. The cover helps prevent polluted wastewater and other objects from falling into the well. It also makes the well safer for children and provides a clean resting place for buckets as people collect water.

The cover should fit neatly over the upper well lining. Clear a flat place to pour a concrete slab and mark out a circle the size of the cover slab to fit the well. Place a ring of bricks around the marked circle. This ring is the slab mold.

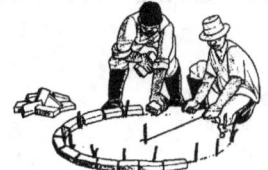

Make a mold for the slab

Leave a hole in the slab for a bucket to pass through or a pump to be fitted. The size of the hole depends on the kind of pump or bucket used, but generally the hole should be large enough for a 10 liter bucket. A can large enough for a bucket to pass through can be used to form the hole.

Place reinforcing wire (3 millimeter) within the slab mold to form a grid with spaces 10 centimeters apart.

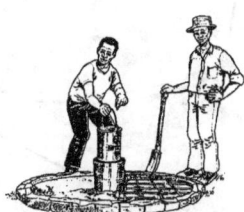

Place reinforcing wire and a mold for the hole

Remove the reinforcing wire grid, and make a concrete mix of 3 parts gravel, 2 parts river sand, and 1 part cement. If stones are not available, use 4 parts river sand and I part cement. Pour concrete in the mold, half way to the top. Place the wire grid on top of the wet concrete. Add the remaining concrete and level with a piece of wood.

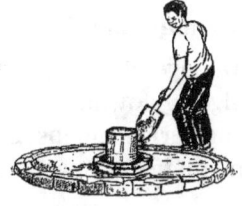

Pour the concrete slab and form the protective collar

Let the slab cure for 1 hour. Remove the bucket hole mold, and fill the central hole with wet sand. Replace the mold on top of the sand and place a ring of bricks around it, leaving 75 millimeters of space between the bricks and the mold. Fill the space between the bricks and the mold with concrete, and let it cure for an hour. After an hour, remove the bricks and the tin mold and shape the protective collar. For the collar to give the best protection, a tin cover should fit snugly over it.

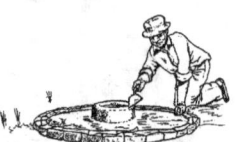

Shape the protective collar

Let the completed slab cure for at least 3 days, keeping it wet the entire time. After it has dried for 7 days or so, place 4 blocks of wood 1 or 2 inches high under the 4 sides of the slab to raise it off the ground. Then dance on it! A well-made slab will not break even with several people dancing on it. Place a bed of cement mortar on the lip of the well lining and carefully set the well cover in place. Keep it covered or shaded for 3 days to prevent the mortar from cracking in the sun.

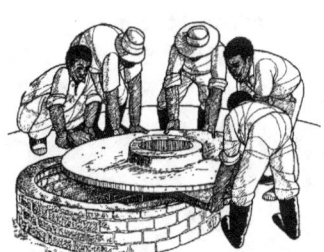

Set the cured well cover in place

The windlass, bucket, and chain

A windlass is a shaft fitted with a handle that makes raising the bucket easier and provides a place to wrap the bucket chain or rope. If a pump is fitted to the well later, the windlass can easily be removed. Attach a durable bucket to the end of the chain or rope. Chain is best because fewer germs will grow on it, but it is costly. Rope is less costly and can be replaced easily if it breaks. Metal buckets will last longer than plastic ones. Durable buckets can be made from used tires and inner tubes.

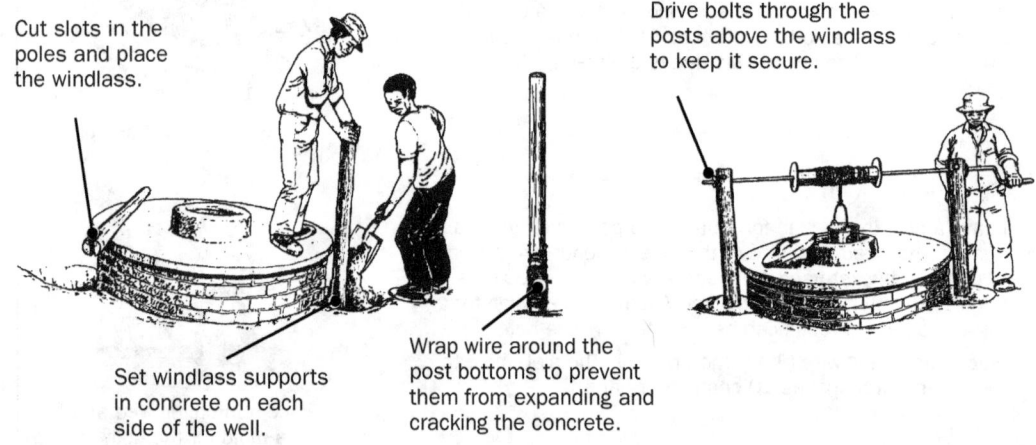

Cut slots in the poles and place the windlass.

Drive bolts through the posts above the windlass to keep it secure.

Set windlass supports in concrete on each side of the well.

Wrap wire around the post bottoms to prevent them from expanding and cracking the concrete.

The drainage platform

The drainage platform carries wastewater and runoff away from the well to a drainage area slightly downhill, to prevent the area around the well from getting muddy and breeding germs and insects. Germs can grow in cracks, so it is important to ensure that the platform is well made.

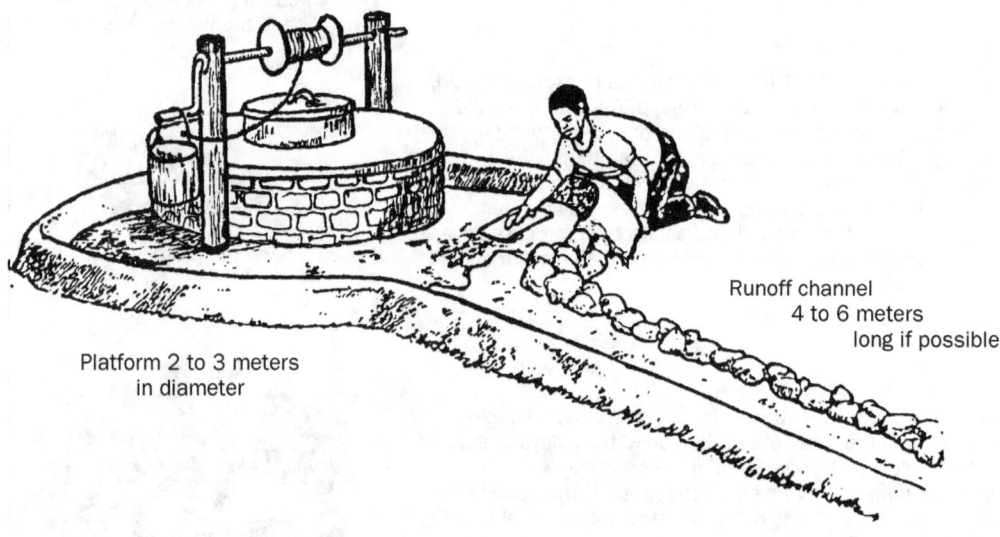

Platform 2 to 3 meters in diameter

Runoff channel 4 to 6 meters long if possible

Pour concrete to a depth of 75 millimeters, with a raised outer rim 150 millimeters high. The entire platform and rim should be reinforced with 3 mm wire to prevent it from cracking.

How to maintain a well

Well water is easily contaminated when dirty buckets and dirty ropes are lowered into the water. Keep one bucket attached to the well and use it to fill other containers. This will ensure the well water stays clean. Providing a way to wash hands before collecting water will also prevent contamination.

- Keep the bucket clean.
- Hang the bucket on the handle of the windlass.
- Keep the well cover in place.
- Always use the same bucket in the well.
- Keep the platform and runoff clean.
- Keep the bucket chain or rope wrapped around the windlass.
- Grease the handle bearing often for ease of use.
- Do not let children play with the well or pump.
- A fence can keep animals out.

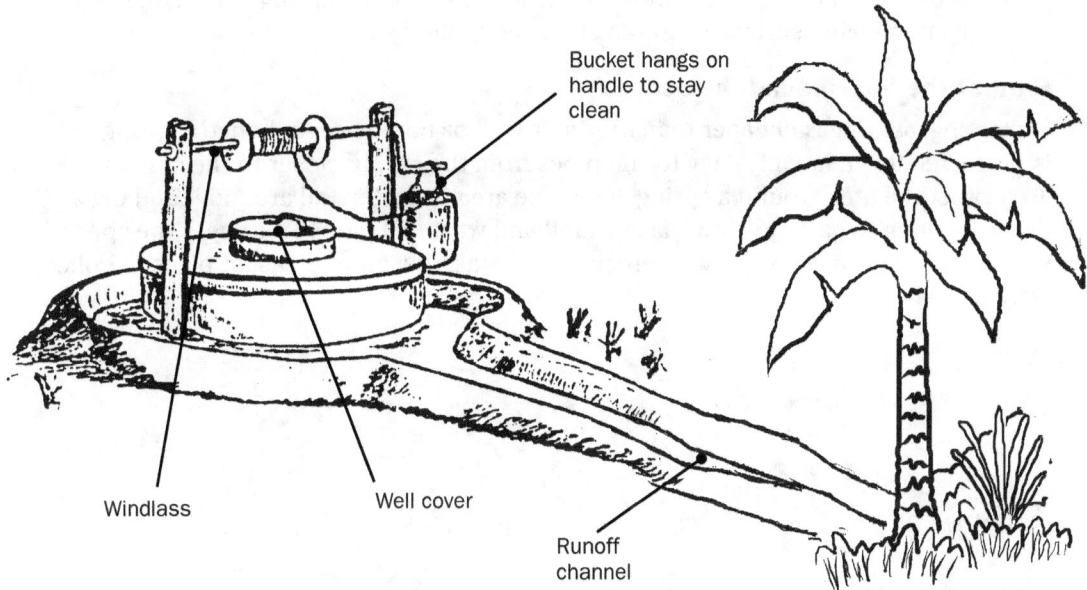

Bucket hangs on handle to stay clean

Windlass

Well cover

Runoff channel

To take advantage of the water that runs off, plant a tree or vegetable garden where the water drains. If you cannot plant a tree or garden, make a hollow in the ground filled with rocks or gravel for the water to seep into. This will also help prevent mosquito breeding.

How to protect a spring

Springs are where groundwater naturally comes to the surface. Because spring water is filtered through rock and soil and is moving quickly, it can be considered safe unless it is contaminated at the surface. To know if a spring is safe, find the true source of the spring — where it comes out of the ground — and ask these questions:

- Is there a stream or other surface water that goes underground above the spring? If so, what appears to be a spring may in fact be surface water that flows a short distance underground. In this case, it will likely be contaminated or may flow only during the rainy season.
- Are there large openings in the rock above the spring? If so, check the water in the spring after a heavy rain. If it appears very cloudy or muddy, contamination from surface runoff is likely.
- Is there a possibility of contamination from human or animal wastes near or just above the source of the spring? This could include pastures for livestock, pit toilets, septic tanks, or other human activity.
- Is the soil very loose or sandy within 15 meters of the spring? This could allow contaminated surface runoff to enter the groundwater.

Protect the area around the spring

Protecting a spring is cheaper than digging a well or borehole. And once a spring is protected it is relatively easy to run pipes from the spring closer to the community. To protect the area around a spring, fence the area 10 meters all around it and dig a drainage ditch to carry away surface runoff and waste. Planting trees near the spring will protect it even more, prevent erosion, and make it a more pleasant place to collect water.

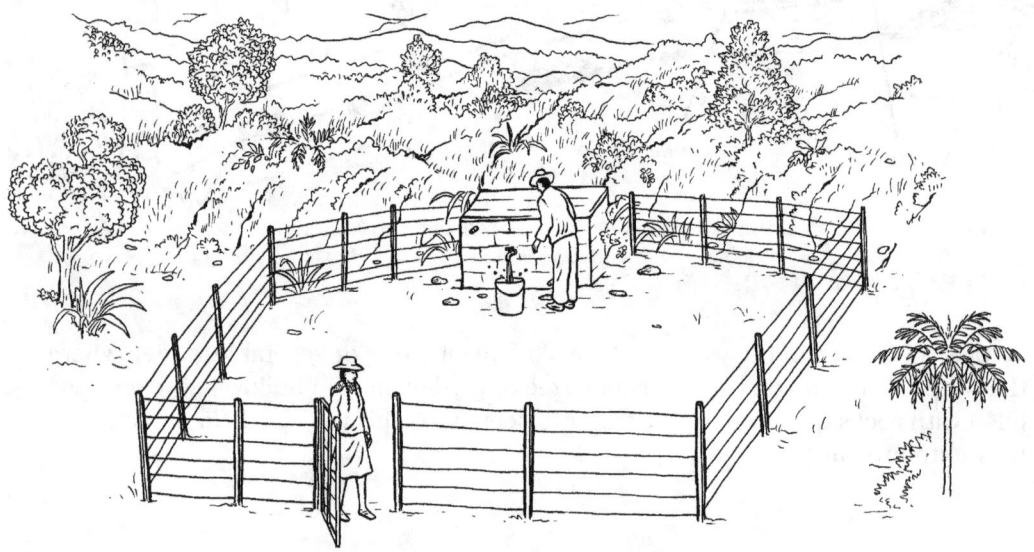

A fence around the spring will keep animals out.

Build a spring box to capture the water

A protected spring should also have a covered *spring box* made of masonry, brick or concrete with an overflow pipe.

Springs may be far from where people live, making water collection difficult. If water is piped from a spring, the spring box built to direct water into pipes may also help protect the water from contamination.

Parts of a spring box

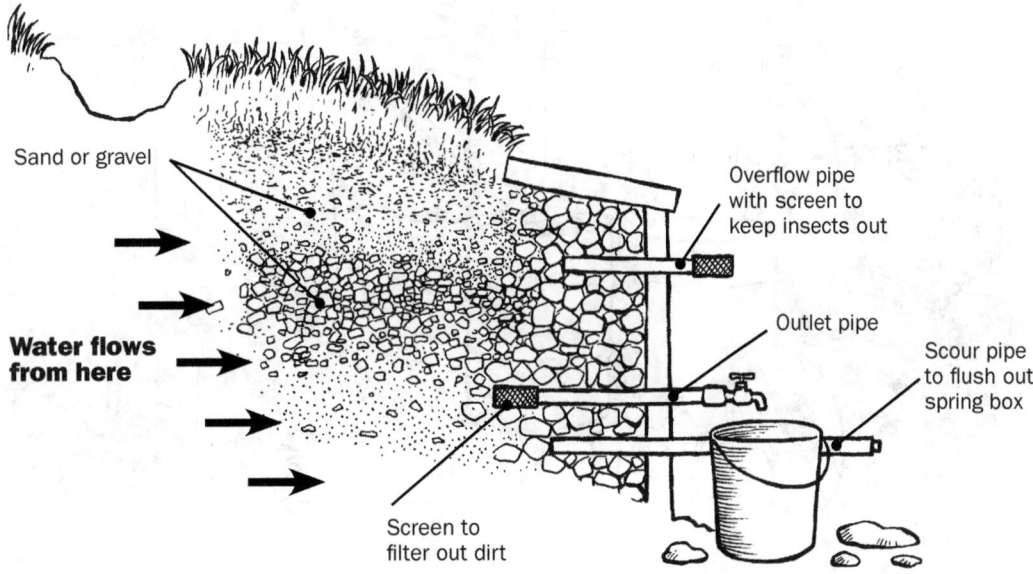

Sand or gravel

Overflow pipe with screen to keep insects out

Water flows from here

Outlet pipe

Scour pipe to flush out spring box

Screen to filter out dirt

This shows a spring box with 1 side cut away to see how the inside looks.

Pipes and spring boxes need cleaning often

Spring boxes need to be monitored to ensure that the spring continues to provide safe water. Silt, leaves, dead animals and other things can collect in the pipes and spring box and block the pipes or contaminate the water. Putting a wire screen on the pipe leading into the spring box will prevent unsafe things from entering pipes. Cleaning the screen every now and again will ensure a steady flow of water.

How to collect rainwater

Harvesting rainwater is one of the safest and most effective ways to collect water. Rainwater is safe to drink except in areas with high air pollution. Rainwater harvesting is a good solution to both water scarcity and water safety.

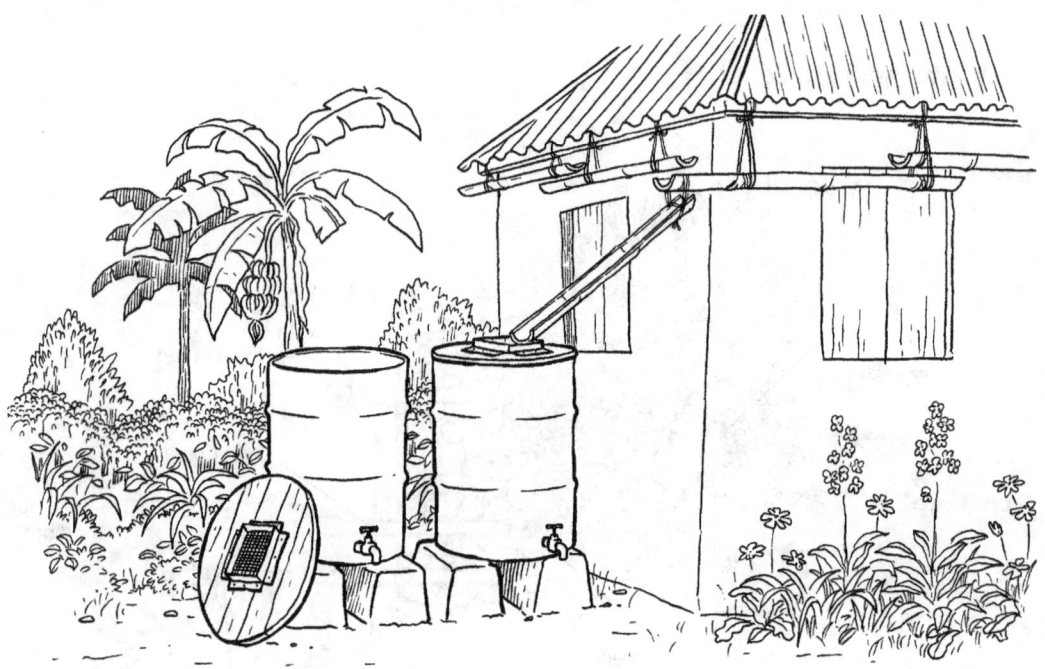

Using a tin roof to collect rainwater.

Rainwater catchments and storage

Above ground tanks can be placed next to the house and the roof will catch rainwater and divert it into the tank. Roofs made of tin or corrugated metal may be used for harvesting rainwater. Roofs made of thatch may collect too much dirt to be safe. Those made of lead or tar have toxic chemicals that make it unsafe to drink the water. Because bird droppings, dead leaves, and dirt collect on roofs, the first rain of the year should be allowed to run off, washing the roof.

Ground catchments can be used to collect surface runoff. A simple reservoir can be made to store water by digging a depression into the ground and compacting the earth or lining it with clay, tile, concrete, or plastic sheeting. These reservoirs can be used to water livestock or to collect water for bathing. If a ground catchment is used for drinking water, it should be fenced to keep animals out. And water used for drinking should be treated using the methods on pages 37 to 43.

Water collected on roofs or in ground level catchments can also be diverted into **underground tanks** for storage. This is a good way to keep water cool. It may also be less costly than building or buying above ground tanks.

How to ensure safe water in a rainwater catchment tank

Collected rainwater must be kept free of contamination to be safe to drink. To ensure that harvested rainwater will be safe:

- Clean the tank and entrance pipe before the rainy season.
- Allow the first rainfall to run through the catchment tank in order to clean it.
- Cover the tank and place a filter or screen over the inlets to keep out insects, leaves, and dirt. This will help prevent mosquitoes from breeding.
- Make sure that water is taken out through taps only, and not by buckets or other containers dipped into the tank.
- For added safety, add chlorine to the tank (see page 41) or connect a water filter to the tank.
- Try not to stir or move the water so any dirt or germs in the tank will stay at the bottom.

Community rainwater harvesting in Rajasthan

Communities in the Thar Desert of Rajasthan, India, have traditionally collected rainwater in many ways. One way rainwater is collected is in village ponds, called *naadi*. Everyone in the village, and even those passing by, may use *naadi* water. In order to protect the water, everyone in the village works to maintain the *naadi*. Ancient laws prohibit any trees from being cut near the edges of the *naadi* or in the area where rainwater collects and runs into the *naadi*. Livestock are kept away from the *naadi,* and people are not permitted to urinate or defecate near it. Once a month, on the day of no moon, the entire village works to dig out sand and silt that has collected in the *naadi*. Digging out the *naadi* makes it deeper and also helps to remove germs that may have settled on the bottom. After digging it out, the villagers allow the water to settle so it becomes clear again. In these ways, the community comes together to protect the precious gift of water.

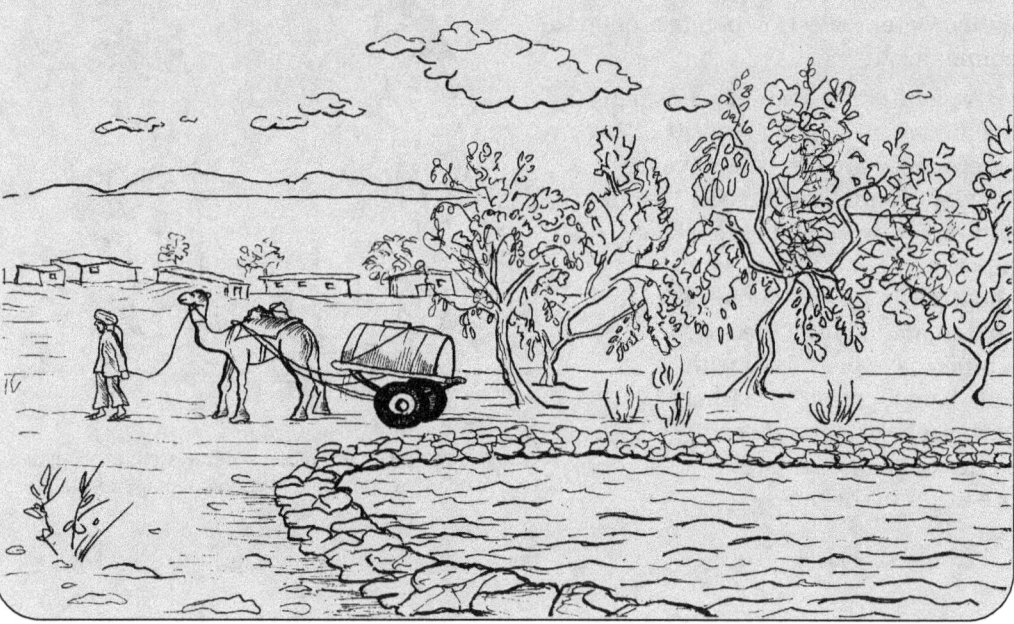

Safe water transport

Transporting water from its source to where people need it is hard work. Care must be taken to keep water uncontaminated while it is being transported.

Carrying water is hard work

Carrying water is some of the hardest work done in any community — and it is often done by women and girls. Carrying heavy loads of water on the back or with a head strap can lead to frequent headaches, backache, malformation of the spine, and can cause a pregnant woman to lose her baby due to strain.

Water improvement projects reduce this burden. Sometimes simple changes can make water carrying easier, water systems can be built to eliminate the need to carry water long distances, or homes can be built closer to the water source. Encouraging men to share this important work will help improve community health.

Piped water

There are many advantages to a piped water system. Piped water reduces the risk of contamination and reduces living places for snails and mosquitoes. A piped water system must be planned carefully, with an understanding of how much water is needed and available, and how much water may be needed in the future as the community grows.

Water can be piped from almost any water source, but springs and reservoirs are most common. The least costly source is one that is uphill from the community, so that gravity will carry the water downhill.

Most piped water systems bring the water to a large storage tank. The tank may be treated with chlorine or have a filter attached to treat the water. Water is piped from the storage tank to tap stands in people's houses or to public water collection points around the community.

A piped water system needs regular maintenance. Keeping records of where pipes are laid can prevent accidents and make it easier to find and repair broken pipes. Leaking pipes can waste a lot of water and draw in sewage and other contamination from the soil. If pipes have been fixed with jute, hemp, cotton or leather, germs may grow on these things and contaminate the water in the pipes.

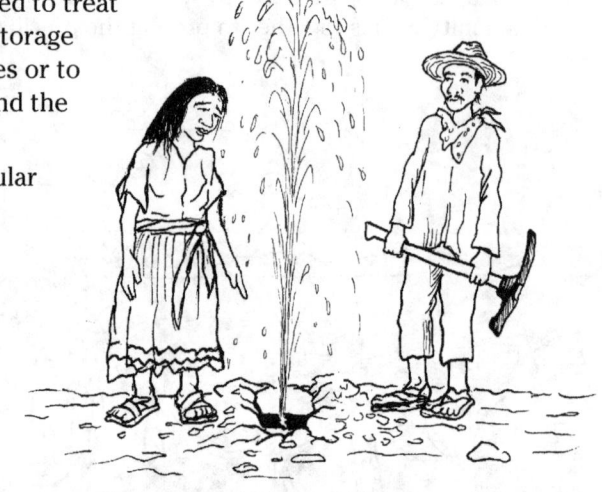

An important part of any piped water system is to ensure that someone is responsible for fixing damage to the pipes.

Women and men work together

When the water committee in a small Mexican village planned to pipe water to the village from a large spring, they decided they had enough money to install a shared tap stand for every 2 houses. At the village assembly the men from the water committee announced that the taps would be used to provide water for drinking and cooking. This was good for the village, they said, because now the women would not spend all day carrying water from the river and boiling it to make it safe to drink.

A woman at the assembly stood up and asked, "What about washing clothes?" One of the men from the water committee said, "You can continue to wash clothes in the river as you always have done." A second woman stood up and asked, "What about bathing our children?" The man said, "You can continue to bathe the children in the river as you always have done." A third woman stood up and asked, "What about our home gardens? We need water to grow vegetables."

The women felt that their voices had not been heard. They said that there was not a single woman on the water committee and so women's needs would not be met. The women demanded that they be allowed to join the water committee and help make a new plan. The rest of the assembly agreed.

The new water committee made a different plan. Rather than a tap for every 2 houses, they would install a tap and a wash basin for every 6 houses. Though they would walk to collect water, they would also be able to wash clothes, bathe children, and clean corn right in the village. The tap stand would be used for drinking water and the washbasin for everything else. This would help ensure that the drinking water stayed clean. And they would use the wastewater from the washbasin to water their home gardens.

The plan was popular among the men as well because it would give them a place to wash their tools when they returned from the cornfields each day. In this way, the villagers met many of their needs at once.

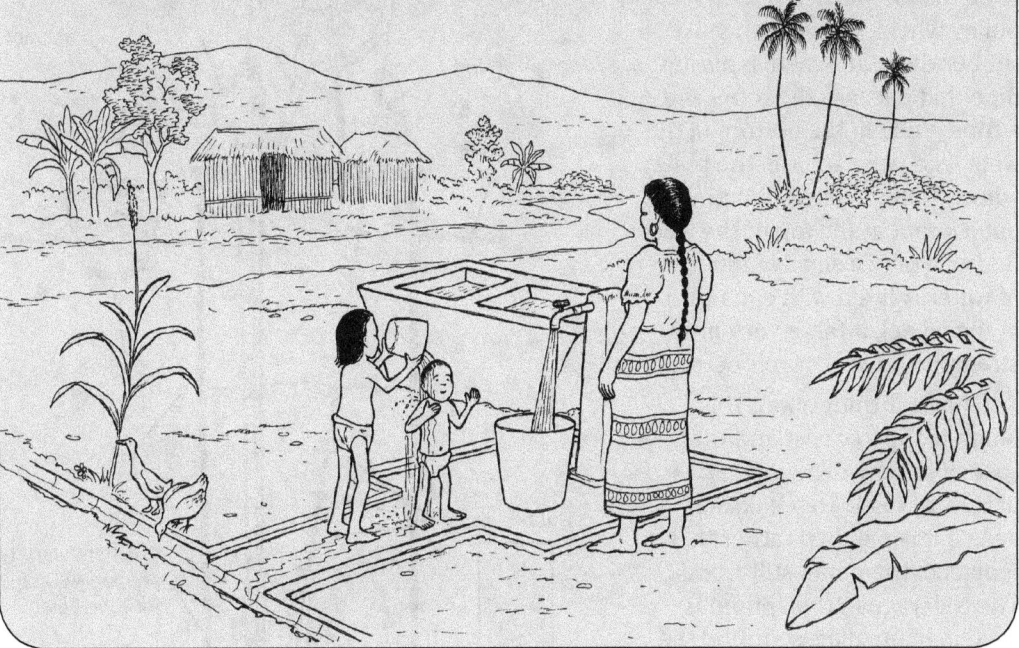

Pumping water from wells

Water flows downhill. A pump is needed to move water uphill. Many kinds of pumps are available including pumps that use electricity, gas, solar energy, or human energy to move water. If a pump is difficult to use or if it is out of service often, people may return to collecting water from unsafe sources.

How to choose a pump

Because a pump may be the most costly part of a water system, it is important to choose the right kind of pump for your household or community. When choosing a pump you may want to consider these things:

- Both men and women should be involved in selecting the community pump.
- A pump should reduce the effort needed to lift water.
- A pump should be manageable by one woman alone.
- A pump should be reliable. If a pump needs costly fuel or electricity which may be unavailable, it is not useful.
- A pump should be easy to repair with available spare parts. A pump that breaks easily but is very easy to repair locally may be better than a pump that will only break after 5 years, but that cannot be easily repaired by local people.

The Nicaraguan rope pump: A low cost, easy way to lift water

All pumps have one thing in common — if they break there is no water. For most people, the best pump is one that they can build, operate, and repair by themselves.

The Nicaraguan rope pump is based on an ancient design from China. It is used to raise water from drilled or hand-dug wells up to 50 meters deep. It uses a metal pulley wheel, a rope with small rubber discs attached, a plastic pipe that encases the rope, and a rope guide in the bottom of the well. As a person turns the pulley wheel, water is lifted and pours out a spout at the top of the well. Because only a small amount of water is lifted with each turn of the wheel, it takes very little strength and is easy to operate.

The best thing about this pump is the low cost and the ease of fixing it. The rope is the part most likely to break, and even if it is patched rather than replaced, the pump still works. The Nicaraguan rope pump is used in many places around the world. In each place people have changed the design to fit their needs and the materials they have to build and repair it.

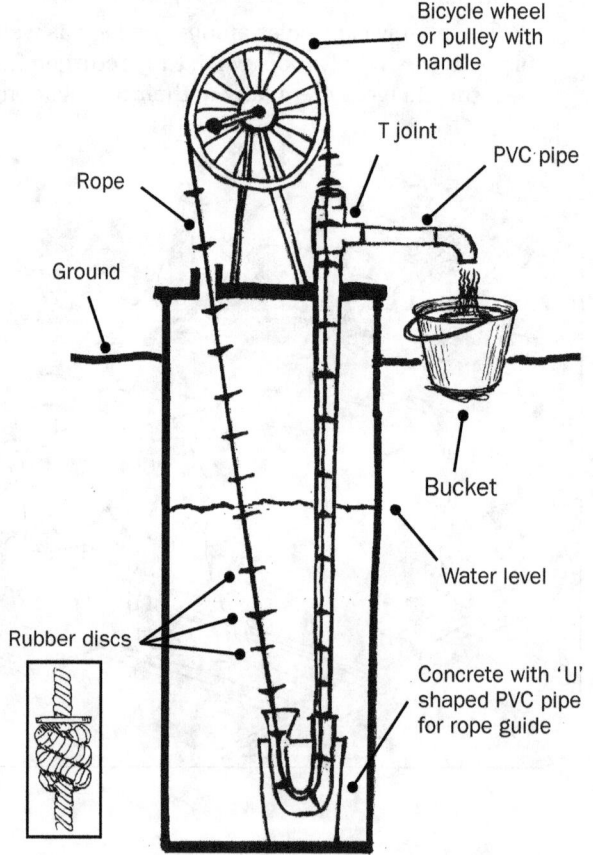

The rope pump is made from low cost, durable parts.

Safe water storage

Water is easily contaminated when it is collected, transported, and while it is stored. To ensure that it is safe, water must be handled carefully while it is being carried and it must be stored in vessels that protect it from further contamination. Water stored in uncovered tanks or tanks with cracked walls, or loose or poorly made covers, is easily contaminated by animal waste and germs. Planning and support of the whole community are necessary to keep water safe for everyone.

SAFE WATER COLLECTION AND STORAGE

This activity helps people think about how water drawn from a well, spring, or tap can become contaminated before it is consumed at home. This activity can be done with any number of people.

 Time: 1 hour

 Materials: Sticky tape, three pictures showing:

1. Two people collecting water at a well, spring, or tap.
2. A child drinking a glass of muddy water
3. Another child drinking a glass of clear water

Step 1: The facilitator shares the picture of the people collecting water with the group. The group discusses what is happening, talking about the people as if they are from this community. What are their names? How often do they collect water? Is the water they are collecting safe? After the discussion, the picture is taped to the wall.

Step 2: The group looks at the picture of the child drinking muddy water. The facilitator explains that this is the child of one of the people from the first drawing, on the next day, drinking the water that was collected. The picture is taped to the wall below the first picture. The facilitator asks, "What happened between yesterday and today to cause the water to become contaminated?" The group discusses all the possible ways the water could have become contaminated.

Step 3: The facilitator shows the picture of the child drinking clear water and tapes it to the wall below the other pictures. She explains that this is the child of the second water collector, and asks, "What has this person done to keep the drinking water clean?" The group then discusses the things that must be done to keep drinking water uncontaminated and how these things can be done in their community and their homes.

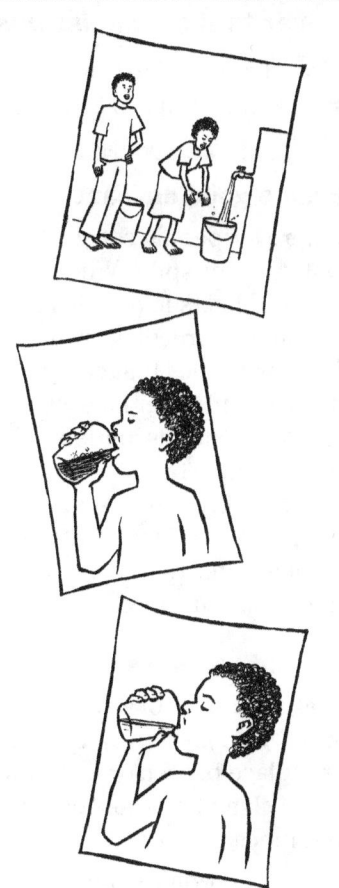

Clean water vessels and keep them clean

Stored water can become unsafe when it is touched by people with dirty hands, when it is poured into a dirty vessel, when dirt or dust gets in the water, and when dirty cups are used. To prevent water from becoming unsafe at home:

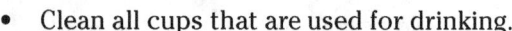

- Wash hands before collecting and carrying water.
- Clean the vessel that is used to carry water.
- Carry water in a covered vessel. This will also prevent spilling.
- Regularly clean the container where water is stored in the house.
- Keep water vessels off the floor and away from animals.
- Pour water out without touching the mouth of the container, or use a clean, long-handled dipper to take water out of the container.
- Clean all cups that are used for drinking.
- Never store water in containers that have been used for pesticides or dangerous chemicals, even if they have been cleaned.
- If possible, do not treat more than you need for daily use, usually less than 5 liters per person per day for drinking and cooking.

Narrow mouthed containers are safest for storing water.

Cover tanks and cisterns

Closed *cisterns* are safer for storing water than open ponds because mosquitoes and snails cannot live in closed tanks. Cisterns should be placed as close as possible to the point of use.

Ensure good drainage

Wherever people collect water, water spills. When water collects in puddles it becomes a breeding ground for mosquitoes that carry malaria and other illnesses. Wells, tap stands, outlets from storage tanks, and other water points should have good drainage that allows spilled water to flow away or to drain into the ground without causing puddles.

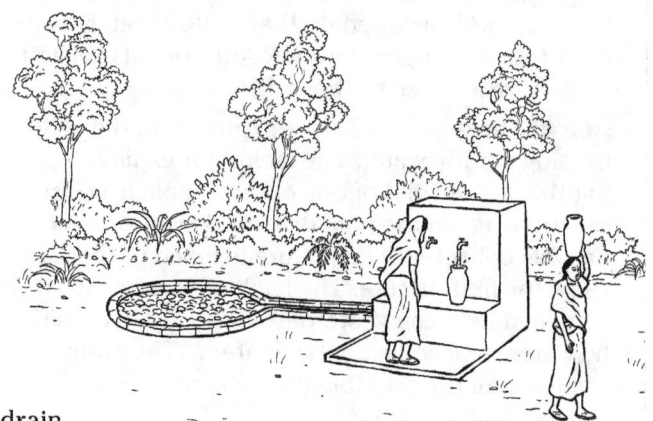

Community water tap with drainage.

Prevent water loss

A large amount of water can be lost through leaks, *evaporation* (when water dries up into the air), and *seepage* (when water soaks into the ground). To conserve water, fix or replace broken or leaky taps, pipes, and tanks as soon as leaks are found. Leaks are also a sign of possible contamination, because germs and dirt enter the cracks in tanks and pipes.

Evaporation can be reduced by covering storage tanks. If water is stored in ponds or ditches, digging them deeper will expose less water to air and so reduce the amount lost to evaporation.

How to make water safe for drinking and cooking

It is better to protect and use a source of safe water than to treat water from a contaminated source, such as a river or water hole. But water will need to be treated if it has been contaminated, if people refuse to drink it due to color or taste, or if it is transported and stored in the home. Water from pipes, tanks, and wells should also be treated before drinking if there is any possibility that it has been contaminated.

The methods you choose to treat water will depend on how much water you need, what it is contaminated with, how you will store it, and what resources are available. **No matter how it is treated it is best to either let the water settle and pour it into another container, or filter the water before disinfecting it.**

The methods shown here do not make water safe from toxic chemicals. **Water with toxic chemicals is never safe for drinking, bathing, or washing clothes.** It may lead to cancer, skin rashes, miscarriages, or other health problems.

To make water safe from germs, follow these steps:

1. Let the water settle for a few hours and pour it into a clean container OR filter it, using

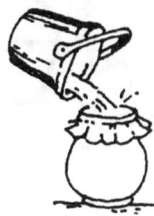

Cloth filter ... or ... **Charcoal filter**

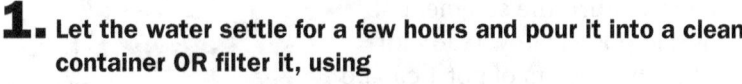

→ Charcoal
→ Thin cloth
→ Sand
→ Pebbles

(See pages 38 to 39 for methods to settle and filter water.)

2. Disinfect the water using **1** of these methods:

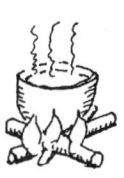 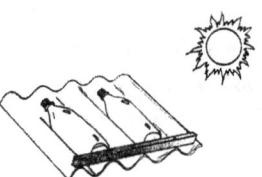 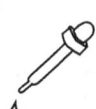 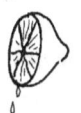

Boiling ... or ... **Solar disinfection** ... or ... **Adding Chlorine** ... or ... **Adding lime or lemon juice**

(See pages 40 to 41 for disinfection methods.)

These basic methods for treating water need little or no equipment. To settle water in ways that take more time but make it safe from most germs, see page 38, Settling water. To learn how to make filters to treat larger amounts of water, see page 43, Ceramic filters, and page 42, Slow sand filters.

Settling water

When water settles, mud, other solids, and germs and worms that cause illness fall to the bottom. Storing water for 5 to 6 days will reduce the number of germs in the water. But some germs, like *giardia*, will not be killed by any length of storage. For this reason it is best to use another method after letting water settle, such as filtering, chlorinating, or solar disinfection.

3 pot method

The 3 pot method settles water so germs and solid matter fall to the bottom. This method is safer than settling water in 1 pot, but it does not make the water completely free of germs. The 3 pot method should be followed by disinfection (see page 40).

Morning, Day 1: Fill pot 1 with water. Cover the top and let it settle for 2 days.

Morning, Day 2: Fill pot 2 with water. Cover it and leave for 2 days. The dirt in pot 1 will begin to settle

Morning, Day 3: Pour the clear water from pot 1 into empty pot 3, making sure not to disturb the sediment at the bottom of pot 1. The water in pot 3 is now ready for drinking. The dirty water left in the bottom of pot 1 can be poured out. Wash pot 1 and refill it with water. Cover it and let it settle for 2 days.

Morning, Day 4: Pour the clear water from pot 2 into pot 3 for drinking. Wash pot 2 and refill it with water.

Morning, Day 5: Pour the clear water from pot 1 into pot 3 for drinking. Wash pot 1 and refill it with water.

Every few days wash the clear water pot (pot 3) with boiling water. If you use a clean flexible pipe to siphon water from one pot to the next the sediment will be less disturbed than if you pour the water.

Using plants to clear and settle water

In many places people use plants to make water safer to drink. One plant used often is *moringa seeds* from East Africa, known as *malunggay* in the Philippines, *horseradish tree* or *drumstick tree* in India, and *benzolive tree* in Haiti and Dominican Republic. To use moringa seeds:

Dry the seeds for 3 days.

Grind the seeds to powder. It takes 15 ground moringa seeds to clear 20 liters of water.

Mix the powder with a little water to make a paste, and add it to the water you want to clear.

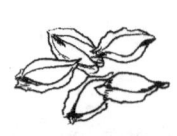

Moringa seeds

Stir for 5 to 10 minutes. The faster it is stirred the less time is needed.

Cover the container and set it aside to let it settle. After 1 to 2 hours, pour the water into a clean container. Be careful to leave the solids in the first container.

Filtering water

There are many ways to filter water to make it safer from germs. Some filters, like the ones on page 42, require special equipment to make, but can filter large amounts of water to make it safe to drink. Other filters, like the ones on this page, require no special equipment and are easy to use to filter smaller amounts of water before disinfecting.

Charcoal filter

This filter is easy to make and works well for removing most germs from small amounts of water. Because the germs that are filtered out will grow on the charcoal, it is important to remove and clean the charcoal often if the filter is used daily, or anytime the filter has been unused for a few days.

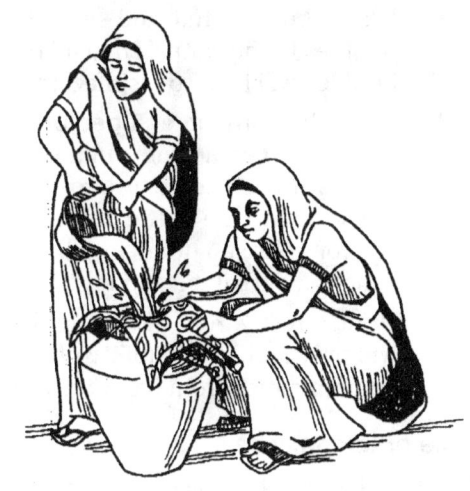

Charcoal
Thin cloth
Sand
Pebbles

1. Punch holes in the bottom of a container with a sharp instrument.
2. Grind charcoal to a fine powder and rinse with clean water. Activated charcoal works best, but ordinary charcoal will work almost as well. NEVER USE CHARCOAL BRIQUETTES! THEY ARE POISON!
3. Place layers of stones, gravel, and sand in the container. Put in a thin cloth and a layer of charcoal on top.
4. Pour water into the filter and collect drinking water from the bottom vessel.

Cloth filters

In Bangladesh and India a filter made of sari cloth, a finely woven cloth, is used to reduce the amount of cholera germs in drinking water. Because the cholera germ often attaches to a tiny animal that lives in water, filtering out these animals also filters out most cholera germs. This method also filters out guinea worms.

You can make a cloth filter out of handkerchiefs, linen, or other fabric. Old cloth is more effective than new cloth because worn fibers make the pores smaller and better for filtering.

1. Let water settle in a container so that solids sink to the bottom.
2. Fold the cloth 4 times and stretch or tie it over the mouth of a water jar.
3. Pour water slowly into the jar through the cloth.

Always use the same side of the cloth, or germs may get into the water. After using the cloth, wash it and leave it in the sun to dry. This kills any germs that may be left in the cloth. In the rainy season, disinfect the cloth with bleach.

Disinfecting water

Disinfecting water kills germs. If done correctly, disinfection makes water completely safe to drink. The most effective methods are boiling, solar disinfection, or using chlorine.

Boiling water

Boiling water for 1 minute makes it safe from germs. Bring water to a rapid, rolling boil. Once it starts boiling, let it boil for 1 full minute before taking the pot off to cool. Water needs to boil for 3 minutes to kill germs in high mountain areas because water boils at a lower temperature high in the mountains.

Boiling changes the taste of the water and boiled water takes a long time to cool, so it cannot be used right away. After boiled water cools pour it into a bottle and shake it strongly. This will add air to the water and improve the taste.

Solar disinfection (SODIS)

Solar disinfection is a very effective way to treat water with only sunlight and a bottle. Filtering or settling the water first will make it clearer so it will disinfect more quickly. Solar disinfection works best in countries close to the equator, because the sun is strongest there. The farther north or south you are, the more time is needed for disinfection to work. (For more information about SODIS see page 47, Where to get more information.)

1. Clean a clear plastic or glass bottle or plastic bag.
2. Fill the bottle ¾ full, and shake it for 20 seconds. This will add air bubbles to the water. Then fill the bottle or bag to the top. The air bubbles will help to disinfect the water faster.
3. Place the bottle in an open place where there is no shade and where people and animals will not disturb it, like the roof of a house. Leave the bottle in the sun for at least 6 hours in full sun, or 2 days if it is cloudy.
4. Drink directly from the bottle. This will prevent the possibility of contamination from hands or other vessels.

Lime or lemon juice

Adding the juice of a lime or lemon to 1 liter of drinking water will kill most cholera and other germs as well. This does not make water completely safe, but may be better than no treatment in areas where cholera is a threat. Adding lime or lemon juice to water before using solar disinfection or the 3 pot method will improve the effectiveness.

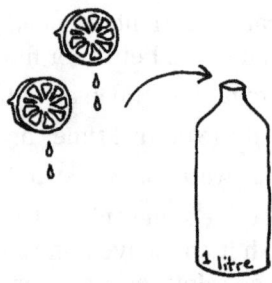

Use 1 lime or lemon for every liter of water.

Chlorine

Chlorine is cheap and easy to use to kill most germs in drinking water. The difficulty with chlorine is that if too little is used it will not kill germs or make the water safe. If too much is used, the water will taste bad and people may not want to drink it.

How much chlorine to add to the water?

The amount of chlorine needed to disinfect water depends on how contaminated the water is (how many and what kinds of germs it contains). The more germs you have, the more chlorine you need to get rid of them. It is important to add enough chlorine so that some is left in the water after the germs are killed. The chlorine that is left is called *free chlorine*. This will kill any new germs that get in the water. If the water has free chlorine in it, it will smell and taste just slightly of chlorine. This tells you it is safe to drink. If it has too much, the smell and taste will be strong and unpleasant.

To use the right amount of chlorine, you need to know how strong your chlorine solution is. Chlorine comes in different forms — gas, bleaching powder, high-test hypochlorite (HTH), and household liquid bleach. Because household bleach is the most common form of chlorine, this book shows how to disinfect water with household bleach.

This booklet shows how to disinfect water with 5% chlorine household bleach. Read the label to see what percentage of chlorine is in your bleach. If it is less than 5%, you will need to add more bleach to the water.

If there is a lot of solid matter in the water the chlorine will be less effective in killing germs. To ensure that chlorine is most effective either filter the water through a cloth or other type of filter (see page 39) or let the water settle so solid matter sinks to the bottom. Pour the clear water off into a clean container and then add chlorine.

WATER		BLEACH	
For 1 liter or 1 quart			2 drops
For 1 gallon or 4 liters			8 drops
For 5 gallons or 20 liter			½ teaspoon
For a 50 gallon or 200 liter barrel			5 teaspoons

Add these amounts of the mother solution to clear water and wait at least 30 minutes before drinking the water. If the water is cloudy, you need twice as much of the bleach solution.

Filters for household and community use

Some filters can provide water that is almost as safe from germs as water that has been boiled, treated by solar disinfection, or treated with chlorine.

Household slow sand filter

This is one of the safest, most effective, and cheapest ways to filter water for a household. This filter can treat at least 50 liters per day — enough for a small family.

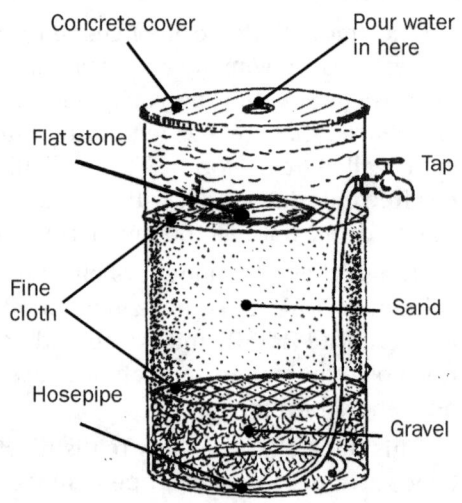

Equipment to make a slow sand filter:

- A watertight container such as a 200 liter barrel, or a large brick or cement jar. Make sure the container did not contain toxic materials
- A 20 millimeter hosepipe with many small holes cut in the first 35 centimeters. This part with holes will lay on the bottom of the barrel.
- A valve or tap
- A small amount of gravel
- Washed river sand
- Fine cloth

HOW TO MAKE A HOUSEHOLD SLOW SAND FILTER

1. Clean the container and disinfect it with bleaching powder.
2. Drill a hole 1/3 of the way down from the top of the container for the tap. The hole should be sized for the fitting on the tap – if the tap has a 12 millimeter fitting, the hole should be 12 millimeters wide.
3. Fit the tap to the hole and fix it in place with hard-setting putty. If a brick container is used, the valve can be cemented within the wall.
4. Prepare the water collecting hosepipe. To do this, drill or punch many small holes in the first 35 centimeters of the hosepipe, seal the end, and form it into a ring on the bottom of the container with the holes facing downward.
5. Connect the water collecting hosepipe to the tap. Seal the pipe fittings with hose clamps or wire.
6. Place a layer of gravel 7 centimeters deep on the bottom of the barrel, covering the water collecting pipe. Cover the gravel with fine cloth and fill the barrel with clean river sand to about 10 centimeters below the tap. Then cover the sand with a second fine cloth.
7. Make a cover for the container, with a hole in it to pour water through. Place a flat rock or dish under the hole to prevent disturbing the sand when water is poured in.
8. Flush the filter with water completely. Once the filter is cleaned, it is ready for daily use.

To use and maintain a slow sand filter

After a few days of use a layer of green scum (bacteria and algae) will grow on top of the sand. This layer helps to treat the water. For this layer to work the sand must always be covered with water. Fill the filter daily and remove water only in small quantities. If the filter is drained completely it will lose its effectiveness, and should be cleaned and refilled.

Every few weeks when water flow from the tap slows down, clean the filter. Let any water out of the filter and remove the green layer and about 1 centimeter of sand from the top. After many cleanings, when more than half of the sand has been removed, replace all the sand and gravel with new cleaned sand and gravel and start over. This may be necessary 1 or 2 times a year.

Improvements to a slow sand filter

Allowing solids to settle out of the water before filtering it will reduce maintenance of the filter because water will be cleaner when it enters. Letting water flow like a waterfall will add air into the water and make it taste better.

A filter has been invented that uses iron nails to filter out arsenic (the arsenic binds to the iron). (To learn about this filter see page 47, Where to get more information.)

Ceramic filters

A small and effective water filter can be made from fired clay coated with colloidal silver (a substance that kills germs). With basic training, a village potter can easily make these filters. (To learn how to produce and promote these filters, see page 47, Where to get more information.)

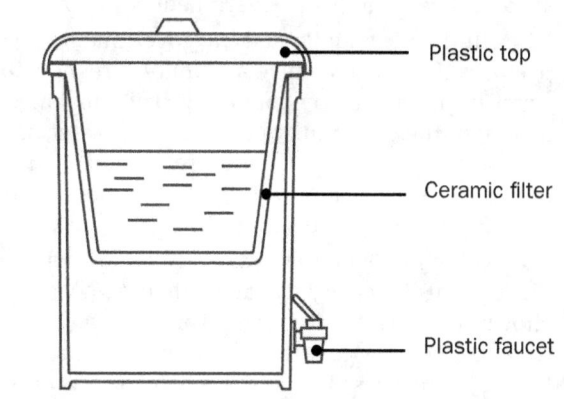

Plastic top

Ceramic filter

Plastic faucet

Ceramic filter used inside a plastic bucket.

Community slow sand filter

Larger filters can be made that connect to surface water sources or piped water systems to supply safe water to a whole village or neighborhood. Where surface water is the only available source, a community slow sand filter is a good way to treat large amounts of water with little work. These filters require an engineer to build and install properly, so we do not describe them here. (To learn more about community slow sand filters, see page 47, Where to get more information, and the International Water and Sanitation Centre.)

Who is responsible for water security?

All over the world people are working to ensure their rights to enough, safe water. Some people believe that private companies can provide better service than governments. But when private companies take control of water services (water privatization), prices are often raised, forcing many people to drastically reduce the amount of water they use. This leads to serious health risks such as diarrhea illnesses. It also forces people to find places where they can collect water for free. This takes a lot of time and hard work, and the water they find may not be safe for drinking.

When governments and communities work together, a good plan to ensure water security — especially for those most in need — can be made.

Partnerships improve water access

In the West African country of Ghana, some community groups have taken the problem of water security into their own hands. In the small town of Savelugu, the government run Ghana Water Company supplies water to the community. The community members are responsible for pricing, distribution, and repair of the water system. They call this a government community partnership.

Both the community and the government run company benefit from the partnership. Because the community is responsible for managing the water, access to water is guaranteed by popular decision making. If some people cannot afford to pay for water, the community pays for their water until they can afford to pay. People's needs are met because they are respected as members of the community — not because they have money to pay. The Ghana Water Company benefits because the community always pays for the water supply.

Savelugu's community based system is being used as a model for small towns throughout Ghana. By managing their own water system, the people of Savelugu have shown that privatization is not the only way to provide water. Since their government community partnership began, there is less illness and everyone has enough water. Their success has shown that community decision making and responsibility is one way to improve water security.

International law and the right to water

Access to enough, safe water is recognized as a human right in many international laws and agreements. One of these agreements, called *General Comment 15*, states:

> The human right to water entitles everyone to sufficient, safe, acceptable, physically accessible and affordable water for personal and domestic uses. An adequate amount of safe water is necessary to prevent death from dehydration, to reduce the risk of water-related disease and to provide for consumption, cooking, personal and domestic hygienic requirements.

Other international agreements that protect the human right to water include:

- The United Nations Charter
- The Universal Declaration of Human Rights
- The Geneva Convention
- The Declaration on the Right to Development
- The Convention on the Rights of the Child
- The Stockholm Declaration
- The Mar del Plata Action Plan
- The Dublin Statement
- Agenda 21
- The Millennium Declaration of Johannesburg
- The European Council of Environmental Law
- Resolution on the Right to Water
- The African Charter on Human and Peoples' Rights
- The Protocol of San Salvador

Most countries have agreed to the conditions of some or all of these conventions. Governments have a responsibility to protect water sources for the common use of all people. Like other rights, the right to water only exists if people use it and defend it. As water grows scarce and becomes a source of ongoing conflict around the world, communities, governments, and international agencies need to work hard to defend the right to water for today and for the future.

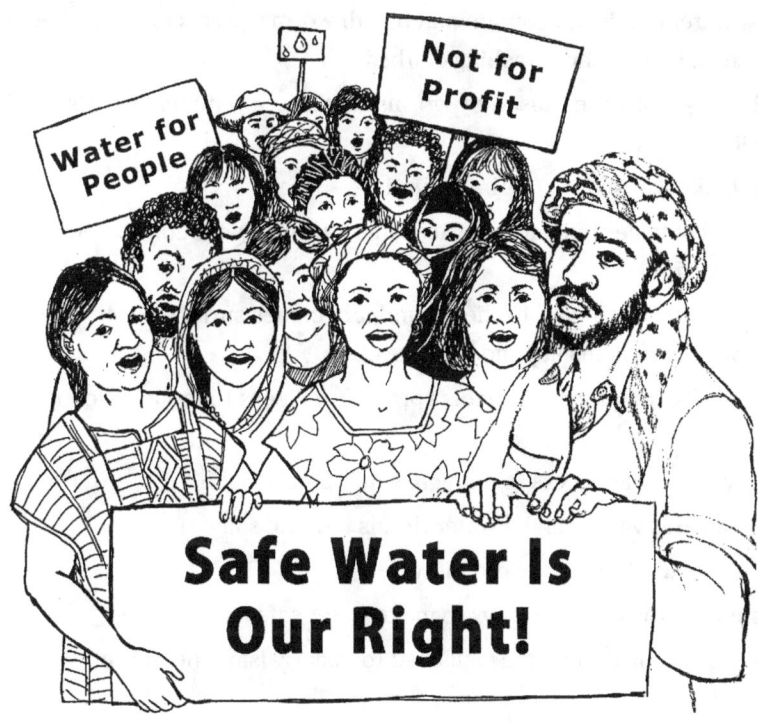

List of difficult words

Accessible — easy to get to.

Algae — very small plants that grow in water and in wet places.

Bacteria — very small organisms that cannot be seen with human eyes. Some bacteria are good and some are harmful for people's health. These are often called germs.

Catchment — an area of land that catches water from rain and small streams and rivers, and sends water downhill into a big river. A catchment is also called a *watershed*.

Chlorine — a chemical used to kill germs and disinfect water.

Cholera — a disease caused by a bacteria that lives in water.

Cistern — a large tank for collecting and storing water.

Conservation — saving the earth's resources from being wasted or destroyed.

Evaporation — when water dries up into the air.

Free chlorine — leftover chlorine that prevents new germs from growing in water that has been disinfected.

Giardia — a parasite that causes yellow, bad-smelling diarrhea, cramps in the gut, and burps that taste like sulfur.

Groundwater — water that flows underground. Groundwater is the source of drinking water in wells and springs. Groundwater may also be called a water table or an aquifer. The groundwater level changes depending on rainfall and how water and land are used.

Guinea worm — a long, thin worm that looks like a white thread. It lives under the skin and makes a painful sore on the ankle, leg, or elsewhere on the body.

Parasite — a tiny animal that lives on — or inside of — our bodies and makes us sick.

Rehydration drink — a drink made of sugar, salt and water or from grain and water that helps retain liquid and restore health when a person is dehydrated.

Safe water — water that is not contaminated with worms, germs or toxic chemicals. It is good for drinking, bathing, and washing clothes.

Schistosomiasis — a disease caused by worms that live in water snails. Also called blood flukes and bilharzia.

Seepage — when water soaks into the ground.

Spring box — a container built at the place where spring water comes above ground, to capture water for drinking.

Surface water — when rain falls to the ground it becomes surface water, where it travels in rivers or streams, or remains in ponds or lakes.

Typhoid — an infection of the gut that is spread from feces to mouth in contaminated food and water.

Water security — regular access to enough, safe water.

Watershed — an area where all the water drains into the same river.

Water table — the top level of the groundwater.

Water treatment — the different ways to make water safe for drinking.

Windlass — the part of a protected well used to make raising the bucket easier.

Where to get more information

For more information about the UNDP's Community Water Initiative see:
http://www.undp.org/water and email contact: *bdp-water@undp.org*

UNDP is involved as a partner organization in the following water-related initiatives which cover various themes including capacity building, governance, and gender:

- Global Water Partnership: *http://www.gwp.org*
- Cap-Net: Capacity Development in Sustainable Water Resource Management: *http://www.cap-net.org*
- World Bank/ Water and Sanitation Program: *http://www.wsp.org/*
- World Water Assessment Programme: *http://www.unesco.org/new/en/natural-sciences/environment/water/wwap*
- Gender and Water Alliance: *http://www.genderandwater.org*
- Hesperian Health Guides: *http://www.hesperian.org*

To contact other water supply programs and organizations worldwide see:

Freshwater Action Network: *http://www.freshwateraction.net*

IRC: supporting water, sanitation, and hygiene services: *http://www.ircwash.org*

Sarar Transformación SC: *http://www.sarar-t.org*

SODIS-Solar Disinfection: *http://www.sodis.ch*

Swiss Resource Center, projects on water supply and sanitation: *http://www.skat.ch/activities/prarticle_view*

WaterAid: *http://www.wateraid.org*

WELL: Resource Centre Network for Water, Sanitation and Environmental Health: *http://www.lboro.ac.uk/well*

World Health Organization (WHO) Water, Sanitation and Hygiene: *http://www.who.int/water_sanitation_health/en*

For a low-cost method to remove arsenic from water, see:
http://web.mit.edu/watsan/Docs/Other%20Documents/KAF/KAF_Construction_Manual_ Jan2006.pdf
for instructions how to build and troubleshoot the Kanchan arsenic filter.

For information about the low-cost ceramic filter, see Potters for Peace:
www.pottersforpeace.com and Email: *pottersforpeace@gmail.com*

Other books from Hesperian Health Guides

Sanitation and Cleanliness, by Jeff Conant and Pam Fadem, offers information on basic sanitation and hygiene, including instructions on building safe, affordable, environmentally-friendly sanitation systems, as well as learning activities to help communities understand and prevent sanitation-related health problems. 48 pages.

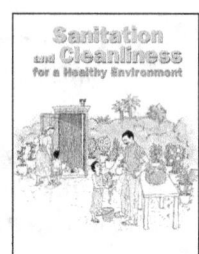

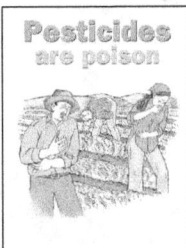

Pesticides Are Poison, by Jeff Conant and Pam Fadem, provides detailed information about pesticides and addresses how to treat people in pesticide emergencies and reduce harm caused by pesticides. It also offers alternate pest control methods that do not use harmful chemicals. 38 pages.

A Community Guide to Environmental Health, by Jeff Conant and Pam Fadem, helps urban and rural health promoters, activists and community leaders take charge of environmental health from toilets to toxics, watershed management to waste management, and agriculture to air pollution. Includes activities, how-to instructions, and stories. 640 pages.

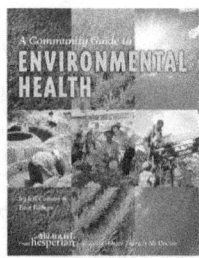

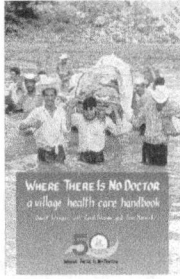

Where There Is No Doctor, by David Werner with Carol Thuman and Jane Maxwell. Perhaps the world's most widely used health care manual, it provides vital, easily understood information on how to diagnose, treat, and prevent common diseases. Emphasizes prevention, including cleanliness, diet, vaccinations, and the role people must take in their own health care. 512 pages.

Where Women Have No Doctor, by A. August Burns, Ronnie Lovich, Jane Maxwell, and Katharine Shapiro, combines self-help medical information with an understanding of the ways poverty, discrimination, and cultural beliefs limit women's health and access to care. Clearly written and with over 1000 drawings, this book is an essential resource for any woman who wants to improve her health, and for health workers who want more information about the problems that affect only women, or that affect women differently from men. 584 pages.

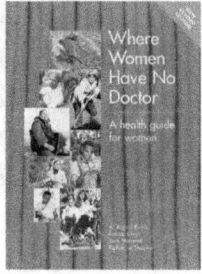

Also available:

Workers' Guide to Health and Safety

Health Actions for Women: Practical Strategies to Mobilize for Change

Recruiting the Heart, Training the Brain: The Work of Latino Health Access

Where There Is No Dentist

A Book for Midwives

Helping Health Workers Learn

Disabled Village Children

Helping Children Who Are Blind

Helping Children Who Are Deaf

A Health Handbook for Women with Disabilities

Learn more about these books at **www.hesperian.org**